Breathing Slower and Less:

The Greatest Health Discovery Ever

Illustrations by Victor Lunn-Rockliffe

Artour Rakhimov

Dr. Artour Rakhimov

Disclaimer

The content provided herein is for information purposes only and not intended to diagnose, treat, cure or prevent cystic fibrosis or any other chronic disease. Always consult your doctor or health care provider before making any medical decisions). The information herein is the sole opinion of Dr. Artour Rakhimov and does not constitute medical advice. These statements have not been evaluated by Ontario Ministry of Health. Although every effort has been made to ensure the accuracy of the information herein, Dr. Artour Rakhimov accepts no responsibility or liability and makes no claims, promises, or guarantees about the accuracy, completeness, or adequacy of the information provided herein and expressly disclaims any liability for errors and omissions herein.

Table of content

Dr. Artour Rakhimov

5

Breathing Slower and Less: The Greatest Health Discovery Ever

Acknowledgments

Let me express my gratitude to all people whose help made the existence of this book possible. In particular, sincere thanks to artist Victor Lunn-Rockliffe (UK) for his beautiful illustrations and to Anne Burns and Mark Callan (Ireland), Steve Green and Carolina Gane (the Netherlands), Ian Pate, Paul Diffley and Duncan Robertson (UK) for proofreading and/or valuable remarks which improved the quality of the manuscript.

I extend my deepest gratitude and heartfelt thanks to my breathing teachers Ludmila Buteyko and Dr. Andrey Novozhilov, MD (both from the Moscow Buteyko Clinic, Russia), and to Victor Lunn-Rockliffe (Great Britain), Dirk van Ginneken (Dutch Buteyko Institute), medical nurse and Glasgow University Lecturer Jill McGowan (Glasgow, Scotland; BIBH), Charles Maguire (Ireland), Peter Kolb (Australia) and many other breathing practitioners and teachers for spiritual support and lively discussions.

Disclaimer

The content provided herein is for information purposes only and not intended to diagnose, treat, cure or prevent cystic fibrosis or any other chronic disease. Always consult your doctor or health care provider before making any medical decisions). The information herein is the sole opinion of Dr. Artour Rakhimov and does not constitute medical advice. These statements have not been evaluated by Ontario Ministry of Health. Although every effort has been made to ensure the accuracy of the information herein, Dr. Artour Rakhimov accepts no responsibility or liability and makes no claims, promises, or guarantees about the accuracy, completeness, or adequacy of the information provided herein and expressly disclaims any liability for errors and omissions herein.

Introduction

The most successful clinical trial in the whole history of cancer research was conducted using the Buteyko method. Dr. Sergey Paschenko, MD, a pupil of Dr. Buteyko, published the results of this trial on 120 people with metastatic cancer (early metastasis) in Ukrainian *Oncology* Journal. The group that practiced reduced breathing exercises had 6 times less mortality in 3 years in comparison with the control group.

Here is another fact: 6 most effective Western clinical trials on asthma were conducted using the Buteyko method. What is common for cancer and asthma? Symptoms and development of these health problems correlates with O2 levels in body cells.

We need more oxygen in body cells to prevent and fight over 150 most popular modern diseases! Yes, modern diseases are virtually always accompanied by low tissue oxygenation. The conditions are ranging from heart disease and cancer, the main killers in the west, to hormonal and digestive problems, diabetes, and asthma.

Tissue hypoxia (low oxygenation of cells) is usually a global phenomenon. No oxygen in one organ or part of the organism usually means that all other vital body organs have inadequate oxygen supply as well. Among them are the brain, heart, kidneys, liver, pancreas, spleen, stomach, both intestines, and hormone producing organs.

Solutions? Oxygen transport depends on many factors, including:
- what and how we eat,
- the way we sleep (sleeping positions),
- posture,
- emotions and stress,
- thermoregulation,

- physical exercise,
- and, of course, the way we breathe.

Should we try to breathe bigger and deeper? Consider the following medical and physiological facts: 1. Take 100 deep and fast breaths through the mouth and you can pass out due to lack of oxygen and blood supply for the brain.

2. Forceful hyperventilation for 15-20 min caused deaths in all dogs and horses due to tissue hypoxia and cardiac failure (heart attack).

3. More breathing means less oxygen and blood for all vital organs (brain, heart, GI organs, liver, lungs, etc.)

4. Sick people (asthma, heart disease, cancer, insomnia, fatigue, etc.) breathe 2-4 times more air per minute than the medical norm.

5. The sicker they are, the faster and deeper they breathe and the shorter their breath holding time (index of oxygenation).

These clinical observations were made by a leading Soviet physiologist Dr. Konstantin Buteyko, MD, PhD. Let us consider these effects, their causes, and clinical evidence in more detail.

Chapter 1. CP (control pause): your oxygenation index

1. 1 You can easily measure your body oxygenation

Breath holding time is an accurate and sensitive measure of tissue oxygenation.

How can we measure breath holding time? We can measure it after exhalation, or after full inhalation, or after 3 or 5 big deep breaths. The test can also be done while sitting or standing. We can also either push the number to its maximum values (hold your breath as much as possible) or stop it at the first signs of air hunger. Out of all these variations, which test is the best representation of oxygenation? Breath holding time after a usual inhalation is greater than after exhalation. The test can also be done after big inhalation. However, one person may have very strong breathing muscles and large capacity of the lungs, another person not.

Hence, parameters of the lungs would affect the results in these cases. What about simple relaxation of the whole body? Such relaxation produces natural spontaneous exhalation. The end of this natural (not forceful!) exhalation is the best time to start the test.

Is it necessary to pinch the nose? Practice shows that, even with our best intentions, we still breathe through the nose when we try to stop breathing but the nose is not pinched. The air exchange is only 5-15% usual breathing, but the results would be less accurate. Hence, we need to pinch the nose (and close the mouth!).

Holding breath for as much as possible is dangerous for many people, for example, due to dramatic increase in blood pressure. Other people can later suffer from panic attacks or migraine headaches due to long breath holds. It would make sense then to stick with a stress-free test, which is done until the first desire to breathe. Practice shows that this first desire appears together with the involuntary push of the diaphragm or swallowing movement in the throat.

(Your body warns you, "Enough!"). If you stop the test and resume breathing at this moment, you will be able to breathe usually or as before the test. No stress, an easy comfortable test.

Look at the diagram below: after the test you can comfortably breathe as before the test.

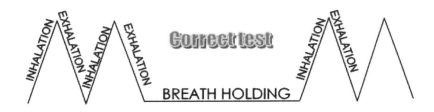

If you hold the breath for too long time, the first inhale will be deep and noisy, as here:

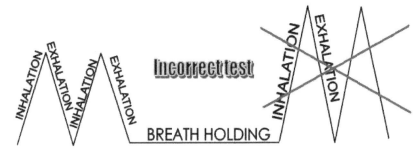

Measurement of the CP (control pause)

Sit down and rest for 5-7 minutes. Completely relax all your muscles, including the breathing muscles. This relaxation produces natural spontaneous exhalation (breathing out). Pinch your nose at the end of this exhalation and count your CP (breath holding time) in seconds. Keep the nose pinched until you experience the first desire to breathe, so that, after you release the fingers, you can resume your usual breathing (in the same way as you were breathing just before you started to hold your breath). Do not extend breath holding too far.

You should not gasp for air or open your mouth afterwards. The test should be easy and must not cause you stress because it does not interfere with your breathing.

1.2 What are the CP norms?

According to the physiological textbook "Essentials of exercise physiology" (McArdle et al, 2000), "If a person breath-holds after a normal exhalation, it takes about 40 seconds before breathing commences" (p.252).

Russian medical Professor Konstantin Buteyko studied oxygenation, breathing and this test for decades. During last four decades, he and his colleagues (over two hundred Russian medical doctors) tested a hundred thousands patients measuring CP many millions times. These health professionals suggested 60 seconds CP, as a value reflecting, among other things, normal tissue oxygenation and absence of many health problems.

1.3 How much are usual CPs when we are sick?

In their studies, breath holding time has been measured by medical people at different phases of breathing (e.g., after normal inhalation, or exhalation, or taking a very deep inhalation, or a complete exhalation). These different conditions can produce large variations in results (by more than 300%).

Moreover, sometimes patients are asked to take 2 or 3 deep breaths before the test. Since researchers use different methods for BHT (breath holding time) measurements, the standardization of results is necessary in order for them to be compared. The explanation of standardization is provided in Appendix 1. All BHT measurements were transformed to the CP as described in this Appendix.

Asthma

A group of American researchers from UCLA School of Medicine found that the breath holding time of asymptomatic asthmatics was less than for normal subjects (Johnson et al, 1995). These (healthy) asthmatics had a CP of about 20 s.

In 1989 Mexican scientists from the National Institute of Respiratory Diseases (Mexico City) found that asthmatics on average had CPs of about 11 s (PerezPadilla et al, 1989). The title of their publication was Rating of breathlessness at rest during acute asthma: correlation with spirometry and usefulness of breathholding time. The researchers found that the breath holding time was a useful (and simple) test that correlated well with the symptoms of asthma.

A group of 14 children with severe asthma, according to a Russian clinical trial, initially had CPs of about 3 s, while 26 children with mild asthma had 5 s CPs in average.

I mentioned above millions of tests done by Soviet and Russian doctors practicing the Buteyko breathing method. They found that between attacks asthmatics usually have about 10-15 s CP, during attacks the CP drops to about 5 s. Symptoms of asthma starts to disappear when the CP is above 20-25 s.

Medical drugs, especially cortical steroids, usually significantly enhance the CP.

Heart disease

Let us look at a study published in 1970 in the Scandinavian Journal of Rehabilitation Medicine (Kohn & Cutcher, 1970). Two American medical doctors from the School of Medicine, State University of New York at Buffalo, New York, conducted thousands of breath holding tests on over 100 cardiac patients. Their tests were done after deep inhalation (with one deep inhale and full exhale before that). This usually results in a time that is about 3 times longer than the CP. Drs. Kohn and Cutcher found the following relationships:

• Functional heart disease (the most severe form) - about 5 s CP;
• Class 2 and 3 heart patients (the moderate and severe forms according to US classification) - about 13 s CP;
• Class 1 heart patients (the light form of the heart disease) - 16 s CP.

These medical professionals concluded that "...an individual unable to hold his breath for at least [7 sec CP] is a poor candidate for vocational rehabilitation".

Moreover, "It is now suggested that the determination of the breath-holding time is an effective screening test for rehabilitation potential" (Kohn & Cutcher, 1970).

In other words, they found that breath holding time test directly relates to the severity of the heart disease. This conclusion is in agreement with the experience of Professor Buteyko, and many Russian and Western Buteyko breathing teachers who often observe the following relationships:
• Heart attacks and strokes - about 5 s CP;
• Severe forms of the heart disease - about 10 s;
• Moderate forms of the heart disease - about 15 s;
• Light forms of the heart disease - about 20 s.

Panic attacks and anxiety disorders

In 1992 clinical Dutch psychiatrists from the State University of Limburg (Maastricht) measured the breath holding time of their patients (Zandbergen et al, 1992). The average CPs were about 11 (for patients with panic attacks) and 16 s (for patients with anxiety disorders).

Canadian scientists from the Department of Psychiatry (University of Manitoba, Winnipeg) found that the average CP of their patients with panic disorders was about 16 s (Asmundson and Stein, 1994).

1.4 The CP: the most accurate parameter of health

According to various Western studies, the CP accurately reflects health and symptoms for asthma, heart disease and many other health problems. In his doctoral thesis, one Russian medical scientist in his PhD showed that the CP was the best and the most accurate single parameter (number) that reflects human health. It is more indicative and more important than heart rate, blood pressure, and any blood test result, ratings of X-ray results, ECG, EEG, and so forth.

1.5 What is the typical CP of people with various diseases?

A typical asthmatic has a CP of approximately 15 s. Obese people and heart patients usually have CPs from 10 to 20 s (10 s for severely sick, 20 with a light degree of disease). During attacks of asthma, stroke, epilepsy, or heart failure, the sufferers have about 5 s CP. There are, however, apparently healthy people who may be free from any organic disease and have a usual CP that is low (down to 10 s or even less).

This chart is based on several Western clinical studies that measured breath-holding abilities in people with various health problems.

Breathing Slower and Less: The Greatest Health Discovery Ever

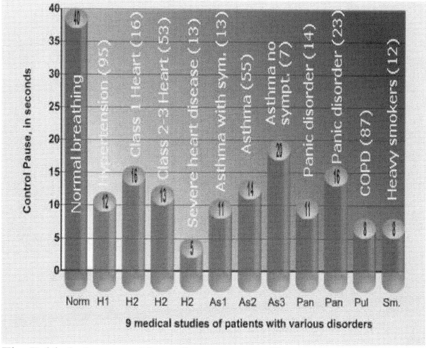

The Table below provides references as well.

Dr. Artour Rakhimov

Condition	Number of subjects	Body Oxygen or Control Pause, s	Reference
Hypertension	95	12 s	Ayman et al, 1939
Neurocirculatory asthenia	54	16 s	Friedman, 1945
Anxiety states	62	20 s	Mirsky et al, 1946
Class 1 heart patients	16	16 s	Kohn & Cutcher, 1970
Class 2-3 heart patients	53	13 s	Kohn & Cutcher, 1970
Pulmonary emphysema	3	8 s	Kohn & Cutcher, 1970
Functional heart disease	13	5 s	Kohn & Cutcher, 1970
Asymptomatic asthmatics	7	20 s	Davidson et al, 1974
Asthmatics with symptoms	13	11 s	Perez-Padilla et al, 1989
Panic attack	14	11 s	Zandbergen et al, 1992
Anxiety disorders	14	16 s	Zandbergen et al, 1992
Outpatients	25	17 s	Gay et al, 1994
Inpatients	25	10 s	Gay et al, 1994
COPD and congenital heart failure	7	8 s	Gay et al, 1994
12 heavy smokers	12	8 s	Gay et al, 1994
Panic disorder	23	16 s	Asmudson & Stein, 1994
Obstructive sleep apnea syndrome	30	20 s	Taskar et al, 1995
Successful lung transplantation	9	23 s	Flume et al, 1996
Successful heart transplantation	8	28 s	Flume et al, 1996
Outpatients with COPD	87	8 s	Marks et al, 1997
Asthma	55	14 s	Nannini et al, 2007

Over 160 Soviet and Russian Buteyko doctors measured the CP in 1,000s of their patients. They got the same general results.

The following relationships generally hold true:
1-10 s - severely sick, critically and terminally ill patients, usually hospitalized
10-20 s - sick patients with numerous complaints and, often, on daily medication
20-40 s - people with poor health, but often without serious

organic problems.
40-60 s - good health
Over 60 s - ideal health, when many modern diseases are
virtually impossible.

These numbers are based on Western research and the practical experience of Russian and Western Buteyko practitioners. There are still many physiological questions and problems. Why is a short CP associated with various diseases? What are the changes in the control of breathing when health improves or deteriorates?

1.6 Can I often measure my CP?

You can make many CP measurements every day. However, some people need to be careful with CP measurements when they have food in the stomach. Breath holding intensifies peristalsis. Many modern western people have some inflammation of the lining of the stomach without being aware about it. Breath holds can make inflammation worse. Be careful after meals! People with panic attacks, heart problems, and migraine headaches may find the test uncomfortable.

However, even without CP measurements one can greatly enhance tissue oxygenation.

1.7 Is the CP stable or very changeable during a day?

If the usual personal CP is very low (about 5-10 s), the CP changes can be as small as a few seconds up or down. In people with larger CPs, the changes can be as large as 10-20 or more seconds. If you measure the CP often, you may realize that it can drop down and recover, but there is a certain range of CP fluctuations and certain maximum value.

The CP can drop, due to, for example, influenza, infection or fever about 2-3 times. You may find that when your CP is low, you have health problems due to acute episodes of your specific condition:

from blocked nose and epilepsy attacks to stroke and bouts of itching.

1.8 What are the main daily factors that influence CP changes?

Meals

The CP drops after meals, especially after overeating (eating when not hungry).

The effect is particularly strong for heavy foods, like animal proteins and fats. If you are not hungry, but still eat such foods, your CP can easily drop 2-3 times.

No wonder, severely sick or old people can die due to one heavy meal. They would rather have many small meals. This prevents deterioration of their health problems.

Self-test. Sometimes you may eat more than you want or eat because of, for example, stress or for social reasons. Measure your CP 2-3 hours after eating when not hungry a heavy meal or overeating. Compare it with your usual CP. How large is the drop? (Do you know that professional marathon runners do not eat any solid or heavy food for 8 hours before important contests?)

Physical activity

During the exercise and soon after, the breath holding time can be short.

However, it is what happens later that matters. The after-effects of physical activity are very different. They depend on personal health and factors related to exercise. For healthy people physical activity is often beneficial. It can be the greatest oxygenation booster and this is one of the reasons why they enjoy physical activity. When we are sick, the effects of exercise are often opposite. The CP after rigorous physical activity can be smaller.

Self-test. On some days you probably have more physical activity than on others. Try measuring your CP just before the exercise. Immediately after the exercise the CP is usually small. However, if you wait about the same time as the duration of the exercise or twice longer, you would be able to see if this exercise was useful for you. Just measure your CP again.

Sleep

When we sleep, one may expect that the CP should become greater in the morning. Why not since sleep is rest? However, this is true only for healthy people or for those who have at least 50-60 s CPs. These people have very short sleep (about 4-5 hours). They wake up having the greater morning CP than the previous evening CP.

For the modern man, the situation is opposite. The unhealthy body, due to abnormal processes and existing physiological stress, depresses tissue oxygenation during sleep. Early morning hours are the times of the lowest CPs. That explains why at the end of sleep (4-7 a.m.), the highest rates of heart and asthma attacks, strokes, and other, often fatal, health problems occur. These are the hours of lowest oxygenation and highest mortality rates.

It is usual that the morning CP is about 10-20 s shorter than the CPs of the previous evening. Sleeping too long further reduces oxygenation. In addition, if one sleeps on the back or breathes through the mouth, the CP drop can be more drastic.

Self-test. If you wake up during the night, check your CP after sleeping in different positions. You need to spend about 15-20 minutes in the same position in order to notice its effects on breathing. Which position suits you best?

Mouth breathing

Breathing through the mouth is a modern health disaster. Nasal breathing warms, humidifies, and cleans the incoming air. Up to 95-99% bacteria, viruses, dust and other air pollutants get trapped on the moist surfaces of the nasal airways. They are designed to be narrow and long. During mouth breathing the irritants and pollutants can travel to bronchi, lungs and blood.

Self-test. If you sometimes keep your mouth open at rest, measure your CP after keeping your mouth open for about 20 minutes. Compare this number with your CP when your mouth is closed after another 20 minute period.

Poor posture

Poor posture (the norm for modern people) also results in reduced CPs.

Practically, slouching means that the CP is below, at least, 25-30 s.

Self-test. Measure your CP when you are relaxed with good posture. Spend 15-20 minutes in an awkward or uncomfortable (e.g., slouching) position with chronically tense muscles. Measure your new CP.

Infections, stress and strong emotions Feeling under stress, having physiological stress (e.g., bacterial or viral infections) and when experiencing many strong emotions cause drop in CPs.

Abnormal thermoregulation

Having extra clothes and being in too warm environment for long time are other factors that interfere with oxygen supply. After 10-20 minutes in such conditions, the CP can decrease by 5-10 or more seconds.

Self-test. Measure your CP in normal conditions. Spend 15-20 minutes in warm or hot conditions. You can do that by wearing more clothes. Check changes in your CP.

All these practical observations produce many questions. Why does overeating reduce oxygenation? Why is sleeping too long, or on the back, or with open mouth dangerous? How does stress hamper oxygenation? These and many other questions have solid scientific explanation. All these effects influence one central factor that directly regulates O2 transport to tissues: the way we breathe. How?

References for Chapter 1

Asmundson GJ & Stein MB, Triggering the false suffocation alarm in panic disorder patients by using a voluntary breath-holding procedure, American Journal of Psychiatry 1994 February; 151(2): p. 264-266.

Ayman D, Goldshine AD, The breath-holding test. A simple standard stimulus of blood pressure, Archives of Intern Medicine 1939, 63; p. 899-906.

Bowler SD, Green A, Mitchell CA, Buteyko breathing techniques in asthma: a blinded randomized controlled trial, Medical Journal of Australia 1998; 169: p. 575-578.

Buteyko KP, Dyomin DV, Odintsova MP, The relationship between lung ventilation and tone of peripheral blood vessels in patients with hypertension and stenocardia [in Ukrainian], Physiological magazine 1965, 11 (5).

Davidson JT, Whipp BJ, Wasserman K, Koyal SN, Lugliani R, Role of the carotid bodies in breath-holding, New England Journal of Medicine 1974 April 11; 290(15): p. 819-822.

Flume PA, Eldridge FL, Edwards LJ, Mattison LE, Relief of the 'air hunger' of breathholding. A role for pulmonary stretch receptors, Respir Physiol 1996 Mar; 103(3): p. 221-232.

Friedman M, Studies concerning the aetiology and pathogenesis of neurocirculatory asthenia III. The cardiovascular manifestations of neurocirculatory asthenia, Am Heart J 1945; 30, 378-391.

Gay SB, Sistrom C1L, Holder CA, Suratt PM, Breath-holding capability of adults. Implications for spiral computed tomography, fast-acquisition magnetic resonance imaging, and angiography, Invest Radiol 1994 Sep; 29(9): p. 848-851.

Johnson BD, Scanlon PD, Beck KC, Regulation of ventilatory capacity during exercise in asthmatics, Journal of Applied Physiology 1995 September; 79(3): p. 892-901.

Kohn RM & Cutcher B, Breath-holding time in the screening for rehabilitation potential of cardiac patients, Scandinavian Journal of Rehabilitation Medicine 1970; 2(2): p. 105-107.

Marks B, Mitchell DG, Simelaro JP, Breath-holding in healthy and pulmonary-compromised populations: effects of hyperventilation and oxygen inspiration, J Magn Reson Imaging 1997 May-Jun; 7(3): p. 595-597.

Mirsky I A, Lipman E, Grinker R R, Breath-holding time in anxiety state, Federation proceedings 1946; 5: p. 74.

Nannini LJ, Zaietta GA, Guerrera AJ, Varela JA, Fernandez AM, Flores DM, Breath-holding test in subjects with near-fatal asthma. A new index for dyspnea perception, Respiratory Medicine 2007, 101; p.246–253.

Perez-Padilla R, Cervantes D, Chapela R, Selman M, Rating of breathlessness at rest during acute asthma: correlation with spirometry and usefulness of breath- holding time, Revistade Investigacion Clinica 1989 July-September; 41(3):p. 209-213.

Taskar V, Clayton N, Atkins M, Shaheen Z, Stone P, Woodcock A, Breath-holding time in normal subjects, snorers, and sleep apnea patients, Chest 1995 Apr; 107(4): p. 959-962.

Zandbergen J, Strahm M, Pols H, Griez EJ, Breath-holding in panic disorder, Comparative Psychiatry 1992 Jan-Feb; 33(1): 47-51.

Chapter 2. Breathing and oxygenation

2.1 What is normal breathing?

Let us start with the international physiological and medical norms for breathing. The man on the left is breathing normally. His breathing is regular, invisible (no chest or belly movements) and inaudible (no panting, no wheezing, no sighing, no yawning, no sneezing, no coughing, no deep inhalations or exhalations). His mouth is closed.

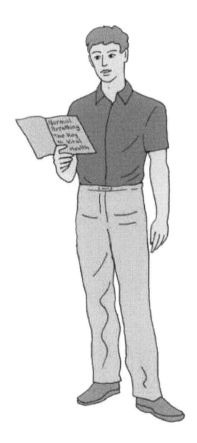

The official medical norm for ventilation is about 6 l/min (liters of air per minute). The main function of breathing is to control concentrations of two gases: CO_2 and O_2.

The corresponding CP is 40 s.

"The perfect man breathes as if he is not breathing" Lao Tze (604 - c.521 BC) Chinese Philosopher

Be observant. If you know people who are healthy (from physiological, social and psychological viewpoints), observe for 1-2 minutes how they breathe at rest. What would you see and hear?

2.2 What is the pattern of normal breathing?

The durations of inhalations and exhalations, breathing rate, amount of air inhaled per breath and other parameters are individual. In addition, they have short- and long-term changes. Some healthy people can have the following parameters of the breathing cycle: inhalation (about 2 s); exhalation (2-3 s); automatic pause or period of almost no breathing (1 s); the depth of inhalation is about 500-600 ml; and breathing rate is about 10-12 times per minute.

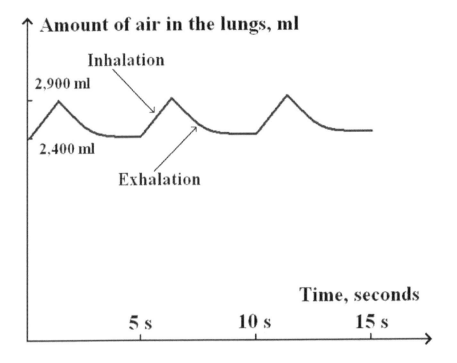

This picture above shows 4 breathing cycles of normal breathing: inhalation (the upward lines), exhalation (the downward lines) and automatic pause (almost the horizontal lines) accompanied by relaxation of all breathing muscles.

As mentioned above, the person with such breathing is going to have about 40 s CP. Most job of inhalation (up to 80-90%) is done by the diaphragm, the main breathing muscle. Exhalation is passive and accompanied by relaxation of all breathing muscles.

2.3 How do sick people usually breathe? They breathe heavily, as in this example on the right.

His breathing is visible (likely chest and belly movements) and audible (possible panting, wheezing, sighing, yawning, sneezing, coughing, deep inhalations or exhalations). His mouth may be open.

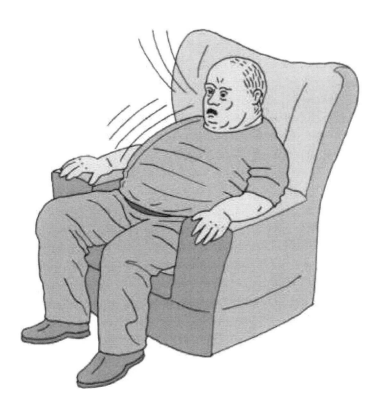

He breathes 12-15 or even more liters of air per minute. He has only 3-5% CO_2 in the lungs and the arterial blood. Most cells of his body are CO_2 and O_2 deficient - heavy breathing makes our cells O_2 deficient, as we are going to learn later.

His CP is less than 20 seconds.

Be observant. Think about and observe those who are ill. What do you see and hear? What happens with your breathing when you are sick or do not feel well?

2.4 What is the typical pattern of breathing of sick people?

For sick people, the durations of inhalations and exhalations, breathing rate, amount of air inhaled per breath and other parameters are very individual. Many sick people can have the following parameters of the breathing cycle: inhalation (about 1.5-2 s), exhalation (1.5-2 s), no automatic pause; the depth of inhalation is about 700-1,000 ml; breathing rate is about 15-20 times per minute.

Breathing Pattern in the Sick

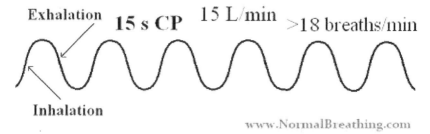

This picture shows several breathing cycles of deep breathing: inhalation (the upward lines) and exhalation (the downward lines). The automatic pause (when breathing movements are absent) is absent.

Note that the exhalation is forceful. Breathing muscles are strained in order to push air out of the lungs. Healthy people, as was shown above, need just to relax all breathing muscles in order to exhale.

Sometimes sick people have an uneven or irregular breathing pattern that includes sporadic sighing, bouts of coughing, periods of fast breathing, etc. All these patterns reduce body oxygenation. They are symptoms of already existing low oxygenation with no more than 30 s CP.

2.5 What happens with the pattern of breathing for terminally ill people and during acute life-threatening episodes?

Most terminally sick people (over 80-90%) have very heavy and deep breathing. They breathe over 20 times per minute taking over 1 liter of air for each breath. Their inhalations and especially exhalations are very short (less than 1.5 s). They need more than 20 l of air for one minute. The CP is about 10 s or less, indicating critically low level of oxygen.

During life-threatening episodes (heart attacks, strokes, asthma attacks, epilepsy attacks, etc.) breathing is even heavier. The CP is only about 5 s.

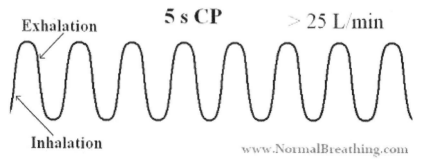

This picture shows several breathing cycles of very deep breathing: inhalation (the upward lines) and exhalation (the downward lines).

2.6 What is the breathing pattern for people with very large CPs?

Excellent breath holding abilities testify for large amounts of oxygen in tissues. Available practical evidence indicates that when people have very large CPs (up to 60-180 s), they have very easy and light breathing pattern at rest. The breathing rate can be only 3-8 breaths per minute with slow relaxed inhalation and long automatic pause (period of no breathing), up to 10 seconds. This corresponds to breathing only 2-4 liters of air per minute. Such CPs indicate absence of many modern health problems.

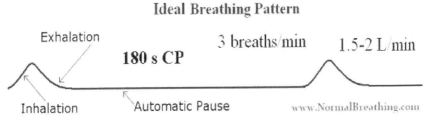

This picture shows 2 breathing cycles of breathing with large CP: inhalation (the upward lines), exhalation (the downward lines) and long automatic pause (the horizontal lines).

Here are all four typical breathing patterns in one diagram.

Breathing patterns and body oxygenation

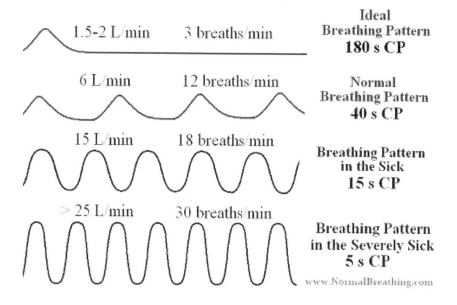

		Ideal Breathing Pattern 180 s CP
1.5-2 L/min	3 breaths/min	
6 L/min	12 breaths/min	Normal Breathing Pattern 40 s CP
15 L/min	18 breaths/min	Breathing Pattern in the Sick 15 s CP
> 25 L/min	30 breaths/min	Breathing Pattern in the Severely Sick 5 s CP

www.NormalBreathing.com

Note. There are, of course, many irregular breathing patterns. Some people sigh every 3-5 minutes. Others cough a lot, or sniff sporadically. Often, breathing through the mouth is a part of the picture. All these irregularities usually are signs of low oxygenation and short CP.

Here we see that deep or/and fast breathing leads to reduced oxygenation of body cells and corresponds to worse health. That's right! The more you breathe, the less oxygen is provided for the cells! If we learn how to have light, shallow, slow and relaxed breathing pattern, oxygenation and the CP will be much higher.

Based on over 40 years of medical research conducted by Russian Medical Professor Konstantin Buteyko and over 200 his medical colleagues, it was found that over 60 s CP is incompatible with many modern health problems. As a result, Professor Buteyko suggested that 60 s CP should be a standard for excellent health.

2.7 How many people have normal breathing?

If we accept medical standards (6 l/min for ventilation, as in most medical and physiological textbooks, and 40 s for the CP), only a small percentage of the population satisfies this criterion. Experience shows that on average, only a few, if any, per 1,000 people have breathing with Professor Buteyko's norm (60 s CP or more).

Most modern people of the West are heavy breathers. They breathe about 8-12 l/min and their usual CPs are about 20-30 s. For sick people the parameters are worse. However, more studies are required to find out the exact extent and prevalence of this problem in the general population of different countries and places.

Be observant. You may ask various people to do the breath holding time test (remember the test should be easy and comfortable). Do you see the correlation between the way the person breathes and his/her CP? What about the CP of sick and severely sick people? How much is your CP when you feel sick, have a cold, flue or infection?

2.8 What is a relationship between ventilation and the CP?

The approximate relationship between ventilation and the CP is linear.

If your CP is 30 s, you breathe twice the norm (about 8 l/min for a 70-kg adult). If your CP is 20 s, you breathe three times the norm (about 12 l/min).

If your CP is 15 s, you breathe 4 times the norm (about 16 l/min).

If your CP is 10 s, you breathe 6 times the norm (about 24 l/min).

Often, you may find that the following practical observations are true. If the chest moves with each inhalation-exhalation cycle (at rest while sitting), then the CP is below 30 s. If, in addition, during breathing the shoulders move, then the CP is below 20 s. Finally, if the head moves, the CP is below 10 s.

2.9 More breathing - less oxygen in tissues!? Why?

During normal breathing (6 l/min for ventilation and 40 s CP), according to numerous physiological textbooks, red blood cells in the lungs become about 98% saturated with oxygen. Breathing more air can slightly increase oxygenation of our lungs. We can get up to 99% blood saturation by heavier breathing. The increase is very small. Do we loose anything? If one starts heavy or deep breathing, the concentrations of CO_2 (carbon dioxide) start to decrease. More CO_2 is removed from the lungs with each breath and therefore the level of CO_2 in the lungs immediately decreases. In 1-2 minutes, the CO_2 level in the blood falls below the normal levels. In 3-5 minutes most cells of the body (including vital organs and muscles) experience low CO_2 concentrations. In 15-20 minutes, the CO_2 level in the brain is below the norm.

Hence, when breathing is heavy all the time, the CO_2 level in all body cells is chronically low. And this is the case with overwhelming majority of sick people. Do we need this gas? Could it be so that CO_2 deficiency causes problems with tissue oxygenation?

"Over the oxygen supply of the body carbon dioxide spreads its protecting wings" 1885, Miescher, a Swiss physiologist

The father of cardio-respiratory physiology, Yale University Professor Yandell Henderson (1873-1944) wrote in his article *Carbon dioxide*,

"But even as early as 1885, Miescher, a Swiss physiologist, in a paper that is one of the masterpieces of physiology, had summarized all the evidence then available and reached the conclusion that it is the variations in the amount of carbon dioxide which principally induce the immediate adjustments of respiration. In a classic phrase inspired by the insight of genius he wrote: Over the oxygen supply of the body carbon dioxide spreads its protecting wings" (Henderson, 1940).

2.10 Greatest health-related superstitions of humanity

Do we need deep or big breathing (also known as over-breathing and hyperventilation)? Should we try to get more fresh air in our lungs so as to improve oxygenation of the cells? Should we try to expel from our bodies, using over-breathing, as much carbon dioxide as possible? Is carbon dioxide a toxic waste and poisonous gas? Most lay people say "yes" to all these questions. However, medically educated people say "no" since they believe that we should breathe very little (that is in accordance with internationally accepted medical and physiological norms). Educated people also believe that we need, for our survival, normal concentrations of carbon dioxide in our blood and cells.

Indeed, there is not a single scientific study that has proven or shown that deep breathing or hyperventilation is useful in normal conditions or at rest. Similarly, there are no studies that have proven or shown that we need to remove as much carbon dioxide as possible. (In fact, a human being will die within minutes if carbon dioxide level drops to a quarter or fifth of the physiological norm.)

At the same time, thousands of professional medical and physiological studies and experiments have proven the adverse effects of acute and chronic over-sbreathing on various cells, tissues, organs and systems of the human organism. Many professional publications confirm the importance of normal carbon dioxide concentrations for various organs and systems in the human body.

Hence, belief in the usefulness of deep breathing (or hyperventilation) is one of the greatest superstitions that exist among the general western population.

2.11 Why CO2 is often considered a "toxic waste and poisonous" gas?

In the 1780s, French scientist Antoine-Laurent Lavoisier determined the composition of air. He also discovered the mechanism of gas exchange during respiration. Oxygen is consumed for the production of energy and carbon dioxide is expelled as an end product. In his classical experiments, mice died in a closed glass jar in an atmosphere containing large quantities of carbon dioxide and almost no oxygen. A candle also quickly expired in such air.

That was probably the time when a superficial understanding of respiration produced the idea that carbon dioxide was "toxic waste and poisonous" gas while oxygen brought life and vigor. "Take deep breath", "Breathe more air, it is good for your health", "Breathe deeper, get more air in your lungs, we need oxygen", etc. became popular phrases for which there is no scientific basis. Even now, some scientific publications contain such misleading sentences, as "Respiration is the process of oxygen delivery."

Professor Yandell Henderson gave the following explanation of this ignorance,

"Likeness of Life to Fire. - Lavoisier's supreme contribution to science and particularly to physiology was the demonstration that, in their broad outlines, combustion in a fire and respiratory metabolism in an animal are identical. Both consist in the union of oxygen from the air with carbonaceous material: and both result in the liberation of heat and the production of carbon dioxide... The human mind is inherently inclined to take moralistic view of nature. Prior to the modern scientific era, which only goes back a generation or two, if indeed it can be said as yet even to have begun in popular thought, nearly every problem was viewed as an alternative between good and evil, righteousness and sin, God and the Devil. This superstitious slant still distorts the conceptions of health and disease; indeed, it is mainly derived from the experience of physical suffering.

Lavoisier contributed unintentionally to this conception when he defined the life supporting character of oxygen and the suffocating power of carbon dioxide.

Accordingly, for more than a century after his death, and even now in the field of respiration and related functions, oxygen typifies the Good and carbon dioxide is still regarded as a spirit of Evil. There

could scarcely be a greater misconception of the true biological relations of these gases... PHYSIOLOGY. -----Relations of Carbon Dioxide and Oxygen in the Body. ---- Carbon dioxide is, in fact, a more fundamental component of living matter than is oxygen. Life probably existed on earth for millions of years prior to the carboniferous era, in an atmosphere containing a much larger amount of carbon dioxide than at present. There may even have been a time when there was no free oxygen available in the air. Even now, such animals as ascaris will live and be active in an atmosphere of hydrogen and entirely without oxygen" (Henderson, 1940).

2.12 What are the primary physiological effects of low CO2?

CO2 was abundant during the evolution of life on Earth. It was part of volcanic gases and was present everywhere in large quantities. Evolutionally, carbon dioxide was as essential for appearance of life as water. It makes sense then that it performs many vital functions in the human body. Here are some of them.

a) CO2 is one of the key players in normal oxygenation of cells due to the Bohr effect

The description of this physiological law can be found in standard physiological textbooks since it was confirmed by dozens of professional studies.

What is the Bohr effect? As we know, oxygen is transported in blood by hemoglobin cells. How do these red cells know where to release more oxygen and where less? Or why do they unload more oxygen in those places where it is more required?

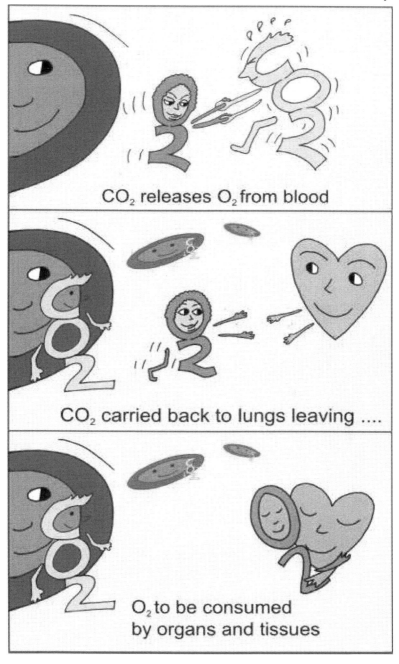

The hemoglobin cells sense higher concentrations of CO_2 and release oxygen in such places. The effect strongly depends on the absolute CO_2 values in the blood and the lungs.

If CO_2 concentration is low, O2 cells are stuck with red blood cells. (Scientists call this effect "increased oxygen affinity to hemoglobin"). Hence, CO_2 deficiency leads to hypoxia or low oxygenation of the body cells (the suppressed Bohr effect).

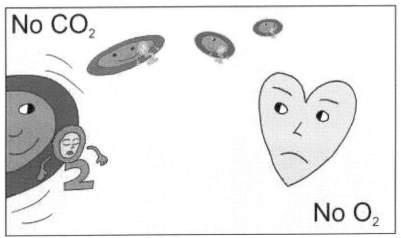

The more we breathe at rest, the less the oxygenation of our cells in vital organs, like brain, heart, liver, kidneys, etc.

Hemoglobin cells in normal blood are about 98% saturated with O2. When we hyperventilate this number is slightly larger, but without CO_2, this oxygen is tightly bound with red blood cells and cannot get into the tissues.

The Bohr effect is crucial for our survival. Why? At each moment of our lives, some organs and tissues work harder and produce more CO_2. These additional CO_2 concentrations are sensed by the hemoglobin cells and cause them to release more O2 in those places where it is most required. This is a smart self- regulating mechanism for efficient O2 transport.

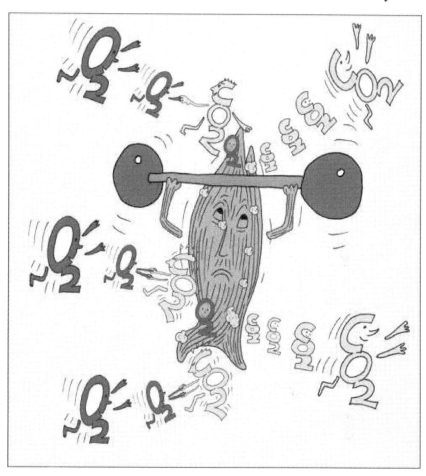

For example, without the Bohr effect, you could not walk or run even for 3-5 minutes. Why? In normal conditions, due to the Bohr effect, more O_2 is released in those muscles, which generate more CO_2.

Hence, these muscles, due to additional oxygen supply, can continue to work with the same high rate.

b) CO_2 is a tranquillizer (or sedative) of all nerve cells

Normal CO2 concentrations create conditions for normal work of the nervous system.

Physiological science accumulated some evidence of adverse effects of low CO2 levels on nerve cells.

Indeed, more than 50 years ago, one of the leading physiological magazines, *Physiological Reviews*, published an extensive research paper, *Physiological effects of hyperventilation*. In this article, American Dr. Brown from the Department of Physiology at the University of Kansas Medical Center analyzed almost 300 professional studies. He stated, *"Studies designed to determine the effects produced by hyperventilation on nerve and muscle have been consistent in their finding on increased irritability"* (Brown, 1953). Muscles and nerve cells become irritated or abnormally sensitive.

Among numerous articles published later, the Journal of Physiology had Cortical CO2 tension and neuronal excitability. It was shown that CO2 has a strong calming effect on excessive excitability of brain areas responsible for conscious thinking (Krnjevic et. al, 1965).

In 1988 physiologists from Duke University (Durham, the UK) suggested in their summary, *"The brain, by regulating breathing, controls its own excitability"* (Balestrino & Somjen, 1988).

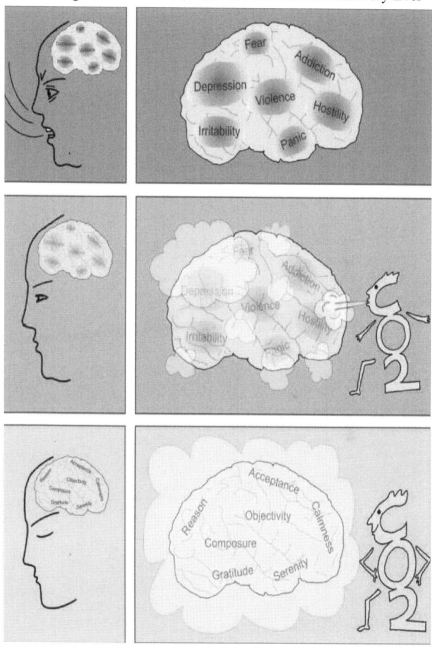

Do modern physiologists have different conclusions? According to a recent study of Finnish scientists from the Laboratory of Neurology

of the University of Joensuu, hyperventilation "*leads to spontaneous and asynchronous firing of cortical neurons*" (Huttunen et. al, 1999). The study was published in *Experimental Brain Research*.

Hence, instead of normal perception, which is characterized by objective reflection and analysis of reality, the brain starts to generate its own "spontaneous and asynchronous" ideas, projects, explanations, and interpretations of real events. Moreover, an excited brain can create problems that, in reality, do not exist.

c) CO2 is a dilator of blood vessels (arteries and arterioles)

Arteries and arterioles have their own tiny muscles that can constrict or dilate depending on CO2 concentrations. At the same time, according to physiological research, the states of these blood vessels are the main factors that define total resistance to blood flow in the body.

Normal breathing and normal arterial CO2 parameters make resistance to blood flow in the cardiovascular system small. Hence, breathing directly participates in regulation of the heart rate.

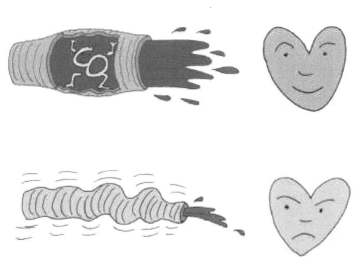

Be observant. When you get a small bleeding cut or a wound, deliberately hyperventilate and see if that can help stop bleeding. It should happen. As an alternative, perform comfortable breath holding and breathe less and accumulate CO_2. What would happen with your bleeding? (It should increase.) Now you know what to do after dental surgeries, brain traumas, and other accidents involving bleeding. It is natural for humans and other animals to breathe heavily in such conditions. Hence, hyperventilation can be life-saving in cases of severe bleeding.

When the CO_2 level is low, total resistance becomes greater and vital organs (like the brain, heart, kidneys, liver, stomach, spleen, colon, etc.) get less blood due to the constriction of small blood vessels. As physiological studies found, blood flow to these organs is proportional to blood CO_2 concentrations.

What about brain blood flow? According to the Handbook of Physiology (Santiago & Edelman, 1986), cerebral blood flow decreases 2% for every mm Hg decrease in CO_2 pressure. When people have 20 mmHg CO_2 in their blood (half of the official norm), they have about 40% less blood supply to the brain in comparison with normal conditions.

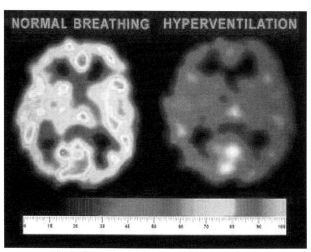

Effects of 1 minute of voluntary
hyperventilation on brain oxygen levels
(vasoconstriction due to a lack of CO_2)

Only some skeletal muscles may get more blood in conditions of hyperventilation.

d) CO2 is a relaxant of all smooth muscles

That was an experimental observation of Dr. Hurlock from the Department of Physiology (University of Birmingham Medical School, UK) in his book Muscle blood flow (Hurlock, 1973).

On the other hand, lack of CO2 makes the muscles tense and irritable. As quoted above, "Studies designed to determine the effects produced by hyperventilation on nerve and muscle have been consistent in their finding on increased irritability" (Brown, 1953).

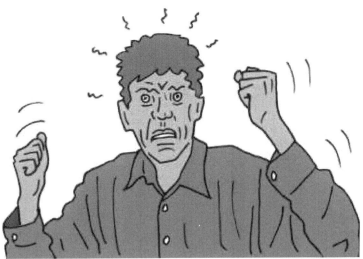

Together with the abnormally excited state of the nervous system, this muscular effect can create conditions of tension and irritability. A slight provocation can create various problems for a hyperventilating person (and for those who are around!) since the muscles are irritated and the brain cells are abnormally excited.

e) CO2 is a natural dilator of bronchi and smaller air passages in the lungs

Normal CO_2 concentrations keep these air passages open wide (see the image below).

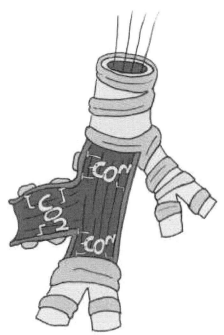

When the CO_2 level in the lungs is low, the bronchi constrict, causing chest tightness, feelings of breathlessness, suffocation and wheezing.

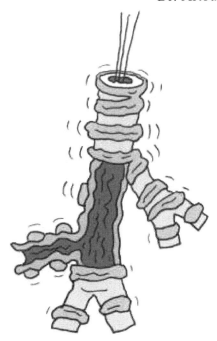

These effects are particularly important for asthmatics.

f) CO2 gas, when dissolved in blood, is the second largest group of negative ions of blood plasma

Hence, breathing directly affects blood pH. In its turn, blood pH is tightly monitored within a very narrow range (from about 7.3 to 7.5) in order to have normal body biochemistry. Therefore, breathing influences concentrations of other ions, including calcium, magnesium, sodium, and potassium, in the blood.

g) CO2 participates in chemical reactions involving various vitamins, minerals, amino acids, essential fatty acids and many other substances

Apart from these effects, the metabolism of proteins, fats and carbohydrates, efficiency of the immune system, regulation of hormones, blood sugar level, and many other chemicals, are all connected to breathing. As a general physiological observation, it has been known for decades that the respiratory system is closely connected with other physiological systems and organs of the organism.

Indeed, all living cells, tissues and organs consume O2 and generate CO2. They breathe -and this process is called the "inner respiration". The outer respiration is the process of breathing. It should make common sense to assume that the way we breathe should influence our inner respiration or cellular gas exchange.

The detailed mechanics of all these interactions are still unknown and here we consider only the most generalized pictures and mechanisms. Moreover, CO2 deficiency is only the most obvious and simple effect of hyperventilation.

Abnormal breathing disrupts, to certain extent, all other systems and fundamental processes in the human body. This CO2-based model, therefore, is only the initial step on the way to understanding human respiration and its role in health and disease.

2.13 When chronically hyperventilating, should I experience all these bad effects?

The above effects are found and should take place in all people. However, the degree of these problems and their personal symptoms (what is felt) are individual. In some people, hyperventilation affects mostly the nervous system, in others cardiovascular, or the respiratory, or the digestive, or the hormonal system, or their combinations. There are people who experience a wide range of negative physiological effects, while some individuals can be less affected. The particular problems depend on genetic make up (or hereditary predisposition) and environmental influences.

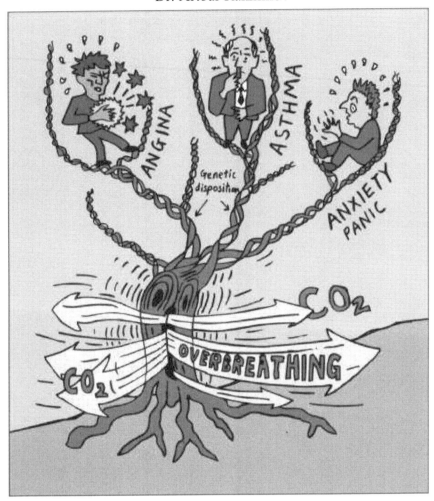

Similarly, the psychological effects of hyperventilation are highly individual and may vary with time for the same person. Indeed, that depends on which over- excited brain area is going to control personal feelings, emotions and behavior.

Physiological research also shows that often it's all in degree. The more we breathe the stronger the effects.

2.14 How do people with diseases react to voluntary hyperventilation?

Yugoslavian doctors from Zagreb asked 90 asthmatics to do voluntary over-breathing (Mojsoski & Pavicic, 1990). All their patients (100%) experienced asthma attacks.

In 1997, the American Journal of Cardiology published results of a similar study performed by Japanese medical professionals from Kumamoto School of Medicine (Nakao et. al, 1997). Over 200 heart patients were asked to hyperventilate, and as you probably guessed, all of them had coronary artery spasms (or symptoms of upcoming heart attacks).

Similarly, people with histories of migraine headaches, panic attacks or epilepsy also experience their specific symptoms. If breathing more can provoke these problems, can it be so that breathing less can prevent them?

2.15 Deliberately heavy breathing can create problems, but does it have any relation to real life?

A large group of French emergency care professionals from Henri Mondor Hospital (Creteil, France) measured the CO_2 level in 120 French patients during non-traumatic cardiac arrest. Their results were published in 1996 in the Critical Care Medicine. The researchers found that *"end-tidal CO_2 could provide a highly sensitive predictor of return of spontaneous circulation during cardiopulmonary resuscitation"* (p.791, Cantineau et al, 1996). The title of the investigation was *End-tidal carbon dioxide during cardiopulmonary resuscitation in humans presenting mostly with asystole: a predictor of outcome.*

In other words, when the heart stops, the CO_2 level can predict the outcome: life or death. (Can CO_2 be a "toxic, waste, and poisonous" gas if it provides life for people suffering a heart attack?)

Note that our cells continuously produce heat due to chemical reactions. The only way to have low CO_2 blood values is by heavy breathing.

More recently a group of ten American doctors from Barnes-Jewish Hospital (St. Louis, USA) tested over 100 patients and wrote an article, End-tidal carbon dioxide measurements as a prognostic indicator of outcome in cardiac arrest (Ahrens et al, 2001). These doctors measured the CO2 concentration in the expired air and this value is usually close to the arterial blood CO2 levels for heart patients. "*CONCLUSION: Measurements of end-tidal carbon dioxide can be used to accurately predict nonsurvival of patients with cardiopulmonary arrest.*" Several other professional studies confirmed these findings.

Does this problem relate only to survival of heart patients? Over 30 years ago the American Journal of Medicine published results of over 8,000 studies of blood gases in a large intensive care unit (Mazarra et al, 1974) where medical professionals and patients literally fought for life. They found that for
15 mm Hg or less CO2 in blood, over-all mortality was 88%
20-25 mm Hg CO2 - 77%
25-30 mm Hg CO2 - 73%
35-45 mm Hg CO2 - 29%.

The conclusion was, "*These findings suggest that extreme hypocapnia [a low level of carbon dioxide] in the critically ill patient has serious prognostic implications and is indicative of the severity of the underlying disease*" (abstract, Mazarra et al, 1974). The names of the most common diseases to occur in all four groups of people were cerebrovascular disease, hepatic coma, bronchopneumonia, and arteriosclerotic heart disease. These are the typical causes of deaths. The title of this investigation was Extreme hypocapnia in the critically ill patient.

Other studies reported the same findings for hepatic coma, bacteraemia, head injuries, heart failure, acute pulmonary infarction, and other common causes of death in modern man.

Note that these studies measured **arterial CO2** which can become abnormally high due to lung damage as in people with COPD (severe asthma, bronchitis and emphysema). However, the cause of lung damage in this people is low CO2 in the lungs: they breathe too heavy and fast; this destroys their lungs and reduces gas exchange in the lungs: the arterial blood carries less oxygen and too much CO_2.

Be observant. Have you seen on TV or in real life how people die? Do you remember how they gasp for air and how these gasps, just before death, become more frantic?

2.16 How is our breathing regulated?

The breathing centre located near the rear of the brain regulates our breathing. The breathing centre (also called the master centre of the body) uses special chemoreceptors to measure CO_2 concentrations in the brain and arterial blood.

The breathing of healthy people during typical daily activities (rest, work, light and moderate exercise, sleeping, etc.) is mainly regulated by the pre-set (or their usual) CO_2 concentrations.

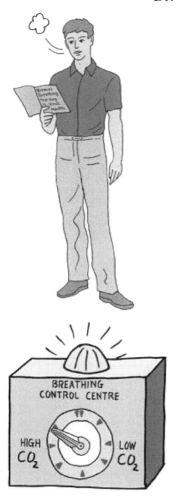

For example, when a healthy person takes several deep and fast breaths, CO2 in the lungs and blood falls. The breathing centre detects this drop and stops the work of the respiratory muscles. The person naturally holds his breath until the CO2 level reaches the initially pre-set value.

Conversely, breath holding accumulates more CO2. The breathing centre senses this increase and intensifies breathing. This over-breathing is going to continue until extra CO2 is removed and the pre-set value is reached.

Breathing Slower and Less: The Greatest Health Discovery Ever

We breathe more heavily during physical exercise, when our bodies produce more CO2. However, the rate of CO2 production matches the rate of CO2 removal in such a fashion that CO2 and O2 values in the arterial blood changes, during exercise, only slightly.

Breathing of sick people is regulated, in addition to CO2, by current arterial blood O2 concentrations.

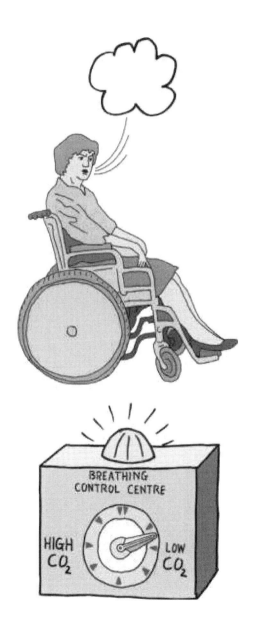

The urge for oxygen gets stronger with advance of many diseases. How and why that happens are some of the least known areas in medicine and physiology.

2.17 Why is it not possible for a sick person to resume normal breathing using will power?

This is another difficult theoretical and physiological question that needs biochemical, neurological, physiological and psychological research. However, a simple explanation is possible. What happens in real life?

Imagine a sick person (e.g., with ventilation 15-20 l/min) who tries to breathe normally (4 or 6 l/min). He/she would quickly accumulate more CO_2 in all cells. That would create a very strong feeling of air hunger (suffocation). It has been found that if a person reduces his minute ventilation about 2 times, he will get a strong air hunger.

Why? One of the known causes is that his/her breathing centre is over-sensitive to additional CO_2. He/she may be able to endure that for some minutes, but not more due to too much stress for the breathing centre. After such a shock and stress of voluntary self-suffocation his/her breathing could get even worse.

Breathing is closely connected with blood flow to all vital organs, sensitivity of the immune system, permeability of cellular membranes, and many other functions. As soon as vital organs (the brain, heart, stomach, kidneys, liver, etc.) are under stress, or inflammation, or injury, breathing gets stronger. That helps to prevent:
- excessive bleeding (as in cases of open injuries, cuts, bruises, etc.),
- quick spread of bacterial and viral infections,
- excessive amounts of toxic products in the blood from injured or polluted tissues,
- damage to vital cleansing organs (e.g., liver and kidneys),
- possible additional damage to the stomach and small intestine due to excessive wear of mucosal surfaces (peristalsis) when CO_2 values get larger.

All these preventive effects can save the life of the organism in the short run. At the same time, it is not normal to be in a state of stress (or fight-flight mode) all the time. Our breathing, if there is no emergency, should be normal.

In order to normalize breathing (or to retrain the breathing centre), all organs and tissues should be gradually repaired, restored and rebuilt. During comfortable and relaxing breathing exercises, a student can reduce his breathing by only about 10-20% in comparison with his initial breathing.

This is a practical conclusion reached by Russian medical professionals practicing the Buteyko method.

2.18 Do people notice their over-breathing (hyperventilation)?

Very rarely. Usually, people notice that their breathing is heavy when they breathe more than 20 or 30 l/min at rest (or 5-7 times the norm!).

Why is this? Air is weightless, and breathing muscles are powerful. During rigorous physical exercise we can breathe up to 100-150 l/min. Some athletes can breathe up to 200 l/min.

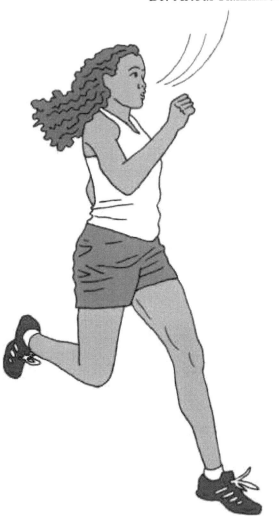

So it is easy to breathe "only" 10-15 l/min at rest, throughout the day and night and not be aware of this rate of breathing. Many people breathe up to 18-20 l/min at rest and claim that their breathing is normal, and does not require many efforts.

It is nevertheless normal during rigorous exercise to breathe, 50 or more l/min since we generate many times more CO_2. As a result, while we are exercising, CO_2 and O_2 concentrations in the arterial blood can remain nearly the same as at rest.

References for Chapter 2

Ahrens T, Schallom L, Bettorf K, Ellner S, Hurt G, O'Mara V, Ludwig J, George W, Marino T, Shannon W., End-tidal carbon dioxide measurements as a prognostic indicator of outcome in cardiac arrest, American Journal of Critical Care 2001 Nov; 10(6): p. 391-398.

Balestrino M, Somjen GG, Concentration of carbon dioxide, interstitial pH and synaptic transmission in hippocampal formation of the rat, Journal of Physiology 1988, 396: p. 247-266.

Brown EB, Physiological effects of hyperventilation, Physiological Reviews 1953 Oct, 33 (4): p. 445-471.

Cantineau JP, Lambert Y, Merckx P, Reynaud P, Porte F, Bertrand C, Duvaldestin P, End-tidal carbon dioxide during cardiopulmonary resuscitation in humans presenting mostly with asystole: a predictor of outcome, Critical Care Medicine 1996 May; 24(5): p. 791-796.

Henderson Y, Carbon dioxide, in Cyclopedia of Medicine, ed. by HH Young, Philadelphia, FA Davis, 1940.

Hurlock O, Muscle blood flow, 1973, Swets & Zeitlinger, Amsterdam.

Huttunen J, Tolvanen H, Heinonen E, Voipio J, Wikstrom H, Ilmoniemi RJ, Hari R, Kaila K, Effects of voluntary hyperventilation on cortical sensory responses. Electroencephalographic and magnetoencephalographic studies, Experimental Brain Research 1999, 125(3): p. 248-254.

Krnjevic K, Randic M and Siesjo B, Cortical CO2 tension and neuronal excitability, Journal of Physiology 1965, 176: p. 105-122.

Mazarra JT, Ayres SM, Grace WJ, Extreme hypocapnia in the critically ill patient, American Journal of Medicine Apr 1974, 56: p. 450-456.

McArdle WD, Katch FI, Katch VL, Essentials of exercise physiology (2-nd edition); Lippincott, Williams and Wilkins, London 2000.

Mojsoski N, Pavicic F, Study of bronchial reactivity using dry, cold air and eucapnic hyperventilation [in Serbo-Croatian], Plucne Bolesti 1990 Jan-Jun; 42(1-2): p. 38-42.

Nakao K, Ohgushi M, Yoshimura M, Morooka K, Okumura K, Ogawa H, Kugiyama K, Oike Y, Fujimoto K, Yasue H, Hyperventilation as a specific test for diagnosis of coronary artery spasm, American Journal of Cardiology 1997 Sep 1; 80(5): p. 545-549.

Santiago TV & Edelman NH, Brain blood flow and control of breathing, in Handbook of Physiology, Section 3: The respiratory system, vol. II, ed. by AP Fishman. American Physiological Society, Betheda, Maryland, 1986, p. 163-179.

Chapter 3. Breathing and modern diseases

Introduction

Which diseases can relate to breathing (or low body oxygenation) and how? Western physiological and medical investigations provide information that supports Professor Buteyko's hypothesis that appearance, development and severity of many common health problems relate to degree of overbreathing.

Each living cell and each living organ of the human body consumes O_2 and generates CO_2. They breathe locally according to their needs and availability of vital nutrients. Would it be logical to assume that their local breathing (inner or cellular respiration) depends on our central breathing (outer respiration)? The modern Western approach to respiration is often based on the following understandings of breathing. "Respiration is the total process of delivering oxygen to the cells and carrying away the by-product of metabolism, carbon dioxide" or "Respiration is the process of taking in oxygen from inhaled air and releasing carbon dioxide by exhalation" or "Respiration is the process by which animals take in oxygen necessary for cellular metabolism and release the carbon dioxide that accumulates in their bodies as a result of the expenditure of energy".

First of all, it is the primary role of breathing to regulate CO_2 (not to release this by-product). Second, while regulation of CO_2 is an important factor, there are many other functions of normal breathing. These other functions can be disturbed. Among frequents abnormalities are: dominance of chest breathing at rest; fast shallow breathing and diaphragmatic flutter; slow inhalations and quick exhalations; periodic breathing; coughing; sighing; and sneezing. These irregularities and infringements are connected with pathological processes or abnormalities in the autonomous nervous system, musculoskeletal system, cardiovascular system, gastrointestinal and other systems of the human organism.

Apart from known CO_2 effects, would it be correct to assume that normalization of breathing can eliminate some pathological processes in other systems of the human body?

3.1 Asthma

Let me mention here that 6 most successful clinical trials on asthma applied the Buteyko breathing method. The goal of this therapy is to slow down breathing to the medical norm. Does this mean that people with asthma breathe too heavy?

In 1968 The New England Journal of Medicine published the results of a large study in which breathing and blood gases of a group of asthmatics were investigated. The researchers found that all 101 tested patients had chronic alveolar hyperventilation. Those asthmatics who had a light or moderate degree of the disease breathed about 15 l of air per min or 2.5 times more than the official medical norm (6 l/min).

More recently, in 1995, American researchers from the Mayo Clinic and Foundation (Rochester) confirmed the same average value (about 15 l/min) for another group of patients diagnosed with asthma (Johnson et al, 1995). This study was published in Journal of Applied Physiology.

Medical professionals from Mater Hospital in Brisbane (Australia) tested 39 asthmatics and found 14 l/min (Bowler et al, 1998), as it was reported in the Medical Journal of Australia.

Each study that measured breathing rates (minute ventilation) in people with asthma found that they breathe about 2-2.5 times more air at rest than the medical norm.

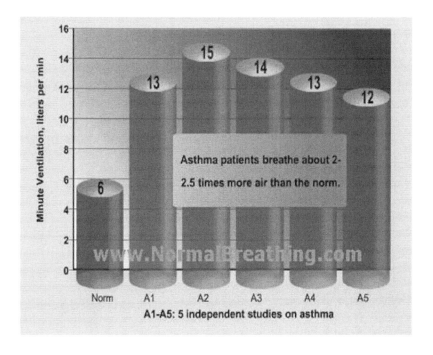

If anyone is interested in more detail and references for these studies, here is a Table.

Minute ventilation rates in asthmatics			
Condition	Minute ventilation	Number of people	References
Normal breathing	6 L/min	-	Medical textbooks
Healthy Subjects	6-7 L/min	>400	Results of 14 studies
Asthma	13 (±2) L/min	16	Chalupa et al, 2004
Asthma	15 L/min	8	Johnson et al, 1995
Asthma	14 (±6) L/min	39	Bowler et al, 1998
Asthma	13 (±4) L/min	17	Kassabian et al, 1982
Asthma	12 L/min	101	McFadden & Lyons, 1968

What evidence exists that low CO2 levels will cause problems with air passages?

Clinical Science published in 1968 an article, The mechanism of bronchoconstriction due to hypocapnia in man ("hypocapnia" means abnormally low CO2 concentrations). In this paper, Sterling explained that CO2 deficiency causes an excited state of the cholinergic nerve. Since this nerve is responsible for the state of the smooth muscles in bronchi, its excited state leads to the constriction of air passages.

What about modern textbooks on physiology? One states, "Agents that tend to dilate airways include increased PaCO2 (hypoventilation or inspired CO2)," (p.545, R. Berne & M. Levy, 1998). This textbook directly claims that slowing down breathing (hypoventilation) or increased CO2 level dilates airways.

Moreover, CO2 is suggested as the chief chemical substance that promotes this effect.

What about the asthma-ventilation connection? Professor Buteyko proposed this link in the 1950's when he discovered the central role of overbreathing in the development and degree of asthma. (He and his colleagues also found that asthma patients got immediate relief from their asthma attack symptoms, if they practiced reduced breathing).

Dr. Herxheimer independently suggested that low CO2 was the cause of bronchial asthma in 1946 and 1952 (Herxheimer, 1946; 1952).

How do asthma and asthma attacks develop? Let us consider the possible mechanism suggested by Professor Buteyko. Low CO2 values in the bronchi cause chronic constriction of airways (that happens in all people). In addition to this direct effect, chronic hyperventilation make immune reactions abnormal. The immune system becomes too sensitive in relation to intruders from outside (coming with air or food), but weakens the responses to various pathogens, like viruses and bacteria. (That makes sense since hyperventilation is a defensive reaction and a part of the flight-or-flight response. Hyperventilation then should mean a state of increased alertness and emergency for the whole organism, the immune system included.) The immune system becomes hypersensitive and seemingly innocent events (like breathing cold air or inhaling dust particles) can trigger an inflammatory response in asthmatics, excessive production of mucus, a sense of anxiety or panic, more hyperventilation, and further constrictions of airways.

As a result, mucus makes air passages narrower (or even blocks some of them) creating a feeling of suffocation and causing asthma attacks. During an attack, an asthmatic may try to clear the mucus by coughing it out, but that further reduces CO_2 concentrations in the lungs and makes air passages narrower.

3.2 Heart disease

Do heart patients over-breathe? In 1995 the British Heart Journal published a study (Clark et al, 1995) done by researchers from the National Heart and Lung Institute in London. The breathing rate of all 88 heart patients at rest ranged from 10 to 18 l/min (or about 2-3 times more than the norm).

In 2000 a study from the Chest magazine a group of American cardiac professionals revealed that patients with chronic heart failure had from 14 to 18 l/min (Johnson et al, 2000).

More recently, Greek doctors from the Onassis Cardiac Surgery Center in Athens recorded ventilation values ranging from 11 to 19 l/min for heart patients from their hospital (Dimopoulou et al, 2001).

There are several other studies with the same conclusion: people with heart disease breathe too heavily.

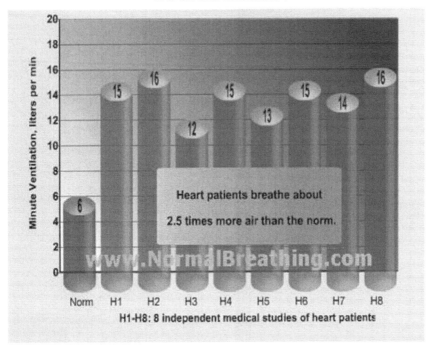

The Table below supplies more detail about these studies.

Minute ventilation rates in heart patients

Condition	Minute ventilation	Number of patients	References
Normal breathing	6 L/min	-	Medical textbooks
Healthy Subjects	6-7 L/min	>400	Results of 14 studies
Heart disease	15 (±4) L/min	22	Dimopoulou et al, 2001
Heart disease	16 (±2) L/min	11	Johnson et al, 2000
Heart disease	12 (±3) L/min	132	Fanfulla et al, 1998
Heart disease	15 (±4) L/min	55	Clark et al, 1997
Heart disease	13 (±4) L/min	15	Banning et al, 1995
Heart disease	15 (±4) L/min	88	Clark et al, 1995
Heart disease	14 (±2) L/min	30	Buller et al, 1990
Heart disease	16 (±6) L/min	20	Elborn et al, 1990

These results raise many questions. Are there any heart patients (with primary hypertension, angina pectoris, and other problems) who have normal breathing parameters? Does the normalization of breathing mean no symptoms and no disease for all people? What are the mechanisms of interactions between breathing and heart disease?

How can hyperventilation affect the heart? Many effects resulting from a CO_2 deficiency can influence the cardiovascular system.

• Low blood CO_2 values lead to **vasoconstriction** or the narrowing of small blood vessels (arteries and arterioles) in the whole body. That causes two problems. First, as a group of Japanese medical professionals found, in conditions of CO_2 deficiency, blood flow to the heart muscle decreases (Okazaki et al, 1991). Hence, heart tissue gets less oxygen, glucose and other nutrients. Second, since small blood vessels are the main contributors to the total resistance in relation to blood flow, CO2 deficiency increases resistance to blood flow and makes the work of the heart harder.

• The **suppressed Bohr effect**, due to low CO2 values in the blood, also reduces oxygenation of the heart muscle. That increases anaerobic metabolism and produces excessive amounts of lactic acid. Note that lactic acid is often implicated as a source of pain in any tissue. In the case of the heart, a person can suffer from angina or chest pain.

• Low CO2 causes **overexcitement of nerve cells in the heart** (the cells that are called pacemakers). This interferes with the normal synchronization and harmony in the working of the heart muscle. (The valves should open and close in proper time, much like a well-tuned engine.). Desynchronization can make the whole process of blood pumping less efficient or more energy- and oxygen-demanding.

• Abnormal metabolism of fats leads, as Russian medical studies revealed, to **increased blood cholesterol level** in some people. That condition gradually, over periods of weeks or months, produces cholesterol deposits on the walls of blood vessels in genetically predisposed people. Such deposits can induce primary hypertension. As their published work suggests, the CP has a linear correlation with the blood cholesterol level.

• Chronic hyperventilation affects the normal work of essential fatty acids causing **changes in inflammatory responses and the malfunctioning of the immune system**.

• Mouth breathing (both at rest and during exercise) is an additional adverse stimulus. It **prevents normal absorption of nitric oxide** (a hormone and powerful dilator of blood vessels) synthesized in the nasal passages.

The father of cardiorespiratory physiology, Yale University Professor Yandell Henderson (1873-1944), investigated some of these effects about a century ago.

Among his numerous physiological studies, he performed experiments with anaesthetized dogs on mechanical ventilation. The results were described in his publication "*Acapnia and shock. - I. Carbon dioxide as a factor in the regulation of the heart rate*". In this article, published in 1908 in the American Journal of Physiology, he wrote, "*... we were enabled to regulate the heart to any desired rate from 40 or fewer up to 200 or more beats per minute. The method was very simple. It depended on the manipulation of the hand bellows with which artificial respiration was administered... As the pulmonary ventilation increased or diminished the heart rate was correspondingly accelerated or retarded*" (p.127, Henderson, 1908).

• Since heart patients breathe 2-3 times more than the official norm, they usually have more frequent and deeper breathing pattern. That must result in other breathing abnormalities, for example, chest breathing, quick inhalations and exhalations. These irregularities indicate **abnormal states of the autonomous nervous and the musculoskeletal systems**.

Which parts of the cardiovascular system are going to be most affected? That depends on genetic predisposition and environmental factors. There are so many factors that can affect the normal work of the cardiovascular system. People are different. Some may get chronic heart failure, others high blood pressure, or stroke, or various abnormalities in the heart muscle.

Do you know that it is possible to get abnormal ECG tracing from a healthy heart just by voluntary heavy breathing? Later, many cardiac professionals, while analyzing such ECGs, can claim pathological changes in the heart. These changes are different in different people. Vice versa, normal breathing naturally eliminates various, already detected, ECG abnormalities.

Modern medicine and physiology has very limited understanding of what is going on with the cardiovascular system when breathing and CO_2 values gradually change in one or the opposite direction. There are many questions related to individual variability, mechanisms of developing pathologies, interaction of hereditary and environmental factors.

3.3 The brain and the central nervous system

What are the main effects of over-breathing on the central nervous system and the brain? Physiology and medicine teach us that a CO_2 deficiency produces the following abnormalities:

• Increased excitability of all nerve cells. We are too excited when we hyperventilate.

• Reduced blood flow to the brain. Our brains get less blood supply. This physiological fact can be found in many textbooks. As Professor Newton from the University of Southern California Medical Center recently reported, "cerebral blood flow decreases 2% for every mm Hg decrease in CO_2" (Newton, 2004). That means that with each second decrease in the CP, blood flow to the brain is less by almost 1%. Less blood means a decreased supply of glucose (the main fuel for the brain in normal conditions), oxygen, and other nutrients. In addition, it causes gradual accumulation of waste products.

• The suppressed Bohr effect. Not only is the inflow of oxygen less, but also its release is hampered by low CO_2 concentrations. That further reduces brain oxygenation.

It is likely that there are other effects of abnormal breathing on the nervous system. Hyperventilation is virtually always manifested in abnormal breathing patterns, including a higher frequency of breathing, shorter exhalations and inhalations, absence of periods of no-breathing, abnormalities in the work of respiratory muscles (e.g., chest breathing), etc. That may cause, for example, the over-activation of sympathetic nervous systems and other negative effects.

Do clinical studies show that patients with mental or psychological problems have heavy breathing?

In 1976 the British Journal of Psychiatry published a study of CO_2 measurements in 60 patients with neurotic depression and non-retarded endogenous depression (Mora et al, 1976). All patients had abnormally low carbon dioxide values.

Later, in 1990, American psychiatrists from Hunter College (City University of New York) reported results from several groups of subjects with anxiety, panic, phobia, depression, migraine, and idiopathic seizures. The abstract states "*virtually all the noncontrol subjects were found to show moderate to severe hyperventilation and accompanying EEG dysrhythmia*". In addition, it notes that hyperventilation and abnormal electrical signals in the brain took place simultaneously.

Canadian scientists from the Department of Psychiatry (University of Manitoba, Winnipeg) measured carbon dioxide concentrations in over 20 patients with panic disorder. Their average CO_2 was also below the medical norm (Asmundson and Stein, 1994). There are many other studies that report abnormally low CO_2 values for people with various psychological and neurological problems.

Is hyperventilation the cause of these health problems?

While these Western studies suggest the possible role of breathing in the appearance and development of various neurological and psychological diseases, modern medicine and psychiatry have a poor understanding of how gradual changes in breathing impact the development of these diseases.

At the same time, there is no any evidence showing that people with normal breathing parameters can suffer from neurological or psychological problems.

3.4 GI (gastrointestinal) problems

How hyperventilation affects the GI system?

• Small blood vessels in the digestive organs get constricted. That reduces their blood supply. Physiological measurements confirm this effect on the stomach, liver, spleen, and the colon. Hence, GI organs get less oxygen, glucose, and other nutrients for their normal work and repair.

• The suppressed Bohr effect, due to low CO_2 values in the blood, reduces the oxygenation of the digestive organs.

• The excited state of the nerve cells in the GI system (the enteric nervous system that orchestrates the normal work of the whole digestive conveyor) interferes with the normal work of the GI organs. That can influence the contraction of the muscular layers, the production and secretion of digestive enzymes and other functions. Indeed, a group of American gastroenterologists from the Mayo Clinic in Rochester recently studied Hyperventilation, central autonomic control, and colonic tone in humans (Ford et al, 1995). They tested the effects of voluntary over-breathing with normal and CO_2-rich air. A drop in the CO_2 level of the blood (hyperventilation) caused abnormalities in the contractility and peristalsis of the colon.

• Chronic hyperventilation can cause autoimmune GI reactions since it is not normal to breathe two-three times the norm 24/7. The immune system, as in case of asthma, can start searching for enemies coming from outside (i.e., with food). This can contribute to the pathology of inflammatory bowel disease, irritable bowel syndrome, Crohn's disease and other problems and complaints.

Hyperventilation can create numerous abnormalities in the GI system. There are no studies that compare these effects or define the individual differences.

Similarly, the impact of permanent changes in breathing (breathing retraining) is also not investigated.

3.5 Cancer

If we compare most successful or most effective clinical trials on people with cancer, it can be a big surprise for most people to find out that the most successful clinical trial in the whole history of cancer research involved application of ... breathing retraining. Dr. Sergey Paschenko, a pupil of Dr. Buteyko, applied the Buteyko method on 120 people with early stages of metastatic cancer. More detail about this stunning victory over early metastatic cancer can be found below.

Let us consider some facts about the appearance, growth and development of malignant tumors; their spread to distant tissues and resistance to standard methods of treatment. What is the abnormal background, which is rarely discussed in popular books and articles about cancer, but which is known to professional oncologists?

What is known about the oxygenation of tissues during the birth and growth of cancer cells or the initial stages of cancer?

It has been known for decades that malignant cells normally and constantly appear and exist in any human organism due to the billions of cell divisions and mutations. These abnormal cells, under normal conditions, are quickly detected by the immune system and destroyed. However, the work of macrophages, enzymes and other agents of the immune system is severely hampered when the conditions of hypoxia exists. That was the conclusion of various studies. For example, Dr. Rockwell from Yale University School of Medicine (USA) studied malignant changes on the cellular level and wrote, "The physiological effects of hypoxia and the associated micro environmental inadequacies increase mutation rates, select for cells deficient in normal pathways of programmed cell death, and contribute to the development of an increasingly invasive, metastatic phenotype" (Rockwell, 1997). The title of this publication is Oxygen delivery: implications for the biology and therapy of solid tumors.

Summarizing the results of numerous studies, a group of biological scientists from University of California (San Diego) chose the following title for their article: The hypoxia inducible factor-1 gene is required for embryogenesis and solid tumor formation (Ryan et al, 1998).

Under normal conditions, even a group of hypoxic cells dies (or is easily destroyed). What about cells in malignant tumors? Researchers from the Gray Laboratory Cancer Research Trust (Mount Vernon Hospital, Northwood, Middlesex, UK) concluded, *"Cells undergo a variety of biological responses when placed in hypoxic conditions, including activation of signaling pathways that regulate proliferation, angiogenesis and death. Cancer cells have adapted these pathways, allowing tumours to survive and even grow under hypoxic conditions..."* (Chaplin et al, 1986).

American scientists from Harvard Medical School noted, that *"... Hypoxia may thus produce both treatment resistance and a growth advantage"* (Schmaltz et al, 1998).

There is so much professional evidence about the fast growth of tumors when the condition of hypoxia is present that a large group of Californian researchers recently wrote a paper *Hypoxia - inducible factor-1 is a positive factor in solid tumor growth* (Ryan et al, 2000). Echoing their paper, a British oncologist Dr. Harris from the Weatherhill Institute of Molecular Medicine (Oxford) went further with the manuscript *Hypoxia - a key regulatory factor in tumor growth* (Harris, 2002).

When the solid tumor is large enough and the disease progresses, cancer starts to invade other tissues. This process is called metastasis. Does poor oxygenation influence it? *"...Therefore, tissue hypoxia has been regarded as a central factor for tumor aggressiveness and metastasis"* (Kunz & Ibrahim, 2003). That was the conclusion of a group of German researchers from the University of Rostock and the University of Leipzig.

Since dozens of medical and physiological studies yield the same result, what about the following title? *Tumor oxygenation predicts for the likelihood of distant metastases in human soft tissue sarcoma* (Brizel et al, 1996). This title claims that tumor oxygenation predicts chances of cancer invasion.

Probably now, the reader can guess about the effect of cancer treatment and the chances of survival for those who suffer from severe chronic hyperventilation. Indeed, "*... tumor hypoxia is associated with poor prognosis and resistance to radiation therapy*" (Chaplin et al, 1986).

"*Low tissue oxygen concentration has been shown to be important in the response of human tumors to radiation therapy, chemotherapy and other treatment modalities. Hypoxia is also known to be a prognostic indicator, as hypoxic human tumors are more biologically aggressive and are more likely to recur locally and metastasize*" (Evans & Koch, 2003).

"*Clinical evidence shows that tumor hypoxia is an independent prognostic indicator of poor patient outcome. Hypoxic tumors have altered physiologic processes, including increased regions of angiogenesis, increased local invasion, increased distant metastasis and altered apoptotic programs*" (Denko et al, 2003).

Could breathing influence the tumors and if so, how? The authors of one of the studies cited above mused about the origins of all these problems, "*Surprisingly little is known, however, about the natural history of such hypoxic cells*" (Chaplin et al, 1986). Why could they appear? What is the source of tissue hypoxia? We can again suggest that our breathing can influence the breathing of all body tissues, tumors included.

What could be the possible chain of events?

Each study that measured various respiratory parameters in people with cancer found abnormal values related to:
- increased respiratory frequency
- increased minute ventilation (or chronic hyperventilation)
- reduced CO_2 levels in the expired air (due to overbreathing).

You can get all these exact numbers with references in my book on cancer. Here is one of the charts reflecting Western clinical evidence.

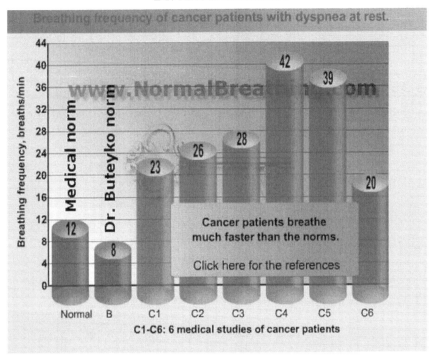

Breathing frequency of cancer patients with dyspnea at rest.

Chronic hyperventilation washes out CO2 from each cell of the human organism. Since CO2 is a dilator of small blood vessels, low CO2 concentrations lead to the constrictions of arterioles causing problems with blood supply and oxygen delivery. In addition, low CO2 values cause inability of red blood cells to release whatever little oxygen they bring (the suppressed Bohr effect). The final outcome is hypoxia in the tissues. This is the necessary background for any cancer. Then genetic and environmental factors can make appearance of tumors in the weakest tissues possible. Further clinical picture depend on interplay of the key parameters: degree of hypoxia, blood and nutrients supply, and other biochemical processes. More research is required to establish the exact chain of events for various conditions.

3.6 Obesity and diabetes

Chronic hyperventilation can develop due to dozens of causes. These causes relate to sleep, exercise, diet and other lifestyle factors that are considered in detail in Chapter 5. However, regardless of these causes, overbreathing usually results in accumulation of body fat. Why does this take place?

When blood vessels are constricted (due to too low arterial CO_2), delivery of glucose to all organs, including the brain, is reduced. Therefore, in order to maintain normal brain function and good wellbeing, most people start to eat more food so as to increase blood glucose levels.

As a result, it is a very common scenario to develop obesity due to overbreathing. Most people who develop hyperventilation start to accumulate extra fat.

However, others may not become obese, but they also suffer from increased blood glucose levels. Both groups of people can be diagnosed with type 2 diabetes mellitus (adult-onset diabetes).

Let us consider clinical research related to minute ventilation at rest in people with diabetes.

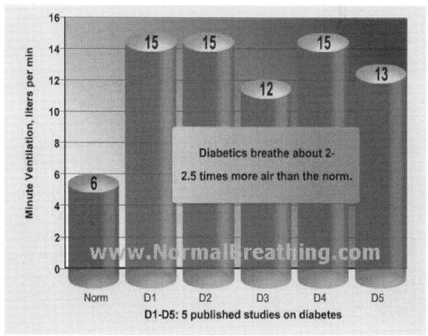

D1-D5: 5 published studies on diabetes

Dr. Artour Rakhimov

More details about these studies are available from this Table.

Minute ventilation rates in diabetics

Condition	Minute ventilation	Number of people	References
Normal breathing	6 L/min	-	Medical textbooks
Healthy Subjects	6-7 L/min	>400	Results of 14 studies
Diabetes	12-17 L/min	26	Bottini et al, 2003
Diabetes	15 (±2) L/min	45	Tantucci et al, 2001
Diabetes	12 (±2) L/min	8	Mancini et al, 1999
Diabetes	10-20 L/min	28	Tantucci et al, 1997
Diabetes	13 (±2) L/min	20	Tantucci et al, 1996

Clinical experience of Russian doctors, as well as my own practical experience, suggests that if a diabetic slows down his or her breathing back to the medical norms (that corresponds to about 40 s CP), then he or she will have normal blood sugar levels naturally or without insulin or medical drugs that reduce blood glucose.

3.7 Other hormonal problems

German endocrinologists from Gutenberg University Hospital (Mainz) tested 42 people with hyperthyroidism and found 15 l/min (Kahaly et al, 1998).

How can deep breathing cause hormonal or endocrine problems?

Since hyperventilation is a state of emergency for the whole body, it can interfere with the normal production and secretion of various hormones. For example, the immediate effects of stress include surges of adrenalin and cortisol. Chronic hyperventilation often leads to deficiencies in these hormones. However, there were no studies that identified the long-range hormonal effects of heavy breathing.

Individual differences and environmental parameters should play their role when it comes to expected effects.

3.8 Other health concerns

What about Western research concerning the breathing of people with various other problems? There were few other studies relating the quality of breathing to other health problems. However, medical science knows little or nothing about the breathing/disease interaction for many common health problems (like cancer, arthritis, diabetes, etc.). That especially relates to the situations when breathing parameters gradually change from one direction to another.

What other diseases are related to abnormal breathing?

Breathing regulates blood supply and oxygenation of all cells, tissues and organs.

Breathing also reflects the state of the autonomous nervous system that regulates the work of all body organs. In conditions of chronic hyperventilation vital organs suffer from reduced blood supply and hypoxia. In addition, chronic hyperventilation interferes with the normal work of the nervous and the immune system. Hence, a wide variety of negative effects is possible when we breathe too much.

Furthermore, if reduced blood and oxygen supply and immune or nervous abnormalities are part of the main problem, then breathing can play a role in further development of this health problem.

Here are studies that we did not quote above. These studies relate to minute ventilation numbers in people with various health problems.

Condition	Minute ventilation	Number of people	All references or click below for abstracts
Normal breathing	6 L/min	-	Medical textbooks
Healthy Subjects	6-7 L/min	>400	Results of 14 studies
Pulm hypertension	12 (±2) L/min	11	D'Alonzo et al, 1987
Cancer	12 (±2) L/min	40	Travers et al, 2008
COPD	14 (±2) L/min	12	Palange et al, 2001
COPD	12 (±2) L/min	10	Sinderby et al, 2001
COPD	14 L/min	3	Stulbarg et al, 2001
Sleep apnea	15 (±3) L/min	20	Radwan et al, 2001
Liver cirrhosis	11-18 L/min	24	Epstein et al, 1998
Hyperthyroidism	15 (±1) L/min	42	Kahaly, 1998
Cystic fibrosis	15 L/min	15	Fauroux et al, 2006
Cystic fibrosis	10 L/min	11	Browning et al, 1990
Cystic fibrosis*	10 L/min	10	Ward et al, 1999
CF and diabetes*	10 L/min	7	Ward et al, 1999
Cystic fibrosis	16 L/min	7	Dodd et al, 2006
Cystic fibrosis	18 L/min	9	McKone et al, 2005
Cystic fibrosis*	13 (±2) L/min	10	Bell et al, 1996
Cystic fibrosis	11-14 L/min	6	Tepper et al, 1983
Epilepsy	13 L/min	12	Esquivel et al, 1991
CHV	13 (±2) L/min	134	Han et al, 1997
Panic disorder	12 (±5) L/min	12	Pain et al, 1991
Bipolar disorder	11 (±2) L/min	16	MacKinnon et al, 2007
Dystrophia myotonica	16 (±4) L/min	12	Clague et al, 1994

There is some limited but encouraging practical evidence about the healing influence of normalization of breathing on a variety of health conditions.

What diseases are not related to chronic hyperventilation? People with, for example, color-blindness lack certain structures in the retina of their eyes. Whatever their breathing patterns, there are no known cases of the appearance or disappearance of this medical condition. Likely, breathing has nothing to do with this problem. Hemophilia is usually manifested in the absence of one blood clotting substance. Again, this problem is purely genetic and probably unrelated to breathing.

There are over 30,000 various health problems and abnormalities known to modern medicine. Professor Buteyko and his Soviet (Russian) medical colleagues, based on their limited clinical experience, hypothesized that about 150-200 health conditions are connected with abnormal breathing. Hence, less than 1% of all health problems might be affected by our breathing. However, many of these health problems are fairly common for modern people. This, for example, relates to our main killers, like heart disease, cancer, and many others.

References for Chapter 3

D'Alonzo GE, Gianotti LA, Pohil RL, Reagle RR, DuRee SL, Fuentes F, Dantzker DR, Comparison of progressive exercise performance of normal subjects and patients with primary pulmonary hypertension, Chest 1987 Jul; 92(1): p.57-62.

Asmundson GJ & Stein MB, Triggering the false suffocation alarm in panic disorder patients by using a voluntary breath-holding procedure, American Journal of Psychiatry 1994 February; 151(2): p. 264-266.

Banning AP, Lewis NP, Northridge DB, Elbom JS, Henderson AH, Perfusion/ventilation mismatch during exercise in chronic heart failure: an investigation of circulatory determinants, Br Heart J 1995; 74: p.27-33.

Bell SC, Saunders MJ, Elborn JS, Shale DJ, Resting energy expenditure and oxygen cost of breathing in patients with cystic fibrosis, Thorax 1996 Feb; 51(2): 126-131.

Bottini P, Dottorini ML, M. Cordoni MC, Casucci G, Tantucci C, Sleep-disordered breathing in nonobese diabetic subjects with autonomic neuropathy, Eur Respir J 2003; 22: p. 654–660.

Bowler SD, Green A, Mitchell CA, Buteyko breathing techniques in asthma: a blinded randomised controlled trial, Medical Journal of Australia 1998; 169: p. 575-578.

Brizel DM, Scully SP, Harrelson JM, Layfield LJ, Bean JM, Prosnitz LR, Dewhirst MW, Tumor oxygenation predicts for the likelihood of distant metastases in human soft tissue sarcoma, Cancer Research 1996, 56: p. 941-943.

Buller NP, Poole-Wilson PA, Mechanism of the increased ventilatory response to exercise in patients with chronic heart failure, Heart 1990; 63; p.281-283.

Buteyko KP, Dyomin DV, Odintsova MP, The relationship between lung ventilation and tone of peripheral blood vessels in patients with hypertension and stenocardia [in Ukrainian], Physiological magazine 1965, 11 (5).

Chalupa DC, Morrow PE, Oberdörster G, Utell MJ, Frampton MW, Ultrafine particle deposition in subjects with asthma, Environmental Health Perspectives 2004 Jun; 112(8): p.879-882.

Chaplin DJ, Durand RE, Olive PL, Acute hypoxia in tumors: implications for modifiers of radiation effects, International Journal of Radiation, Oncology, Biology, Physics 1986 August; 12(8): p. 1279-1282.

Clague JE, Carter J, Coakley J, Edwards RH, Calverley PM, Respiratory effort perception at rest and during carbon dioxide rebreathing in patients with dystrophia myotonica, Thorax 1994 Mar; 49(3): p.240-244.

Clark AL, Chua TP, Coats AJ, Anatomical dead space, ventilatory pattern, and exercise capacity in chronic heart failure, Br Heart J 1995 Oct; 74(4): p. 377-380.

Clark AL, Volterrani M, Swan JW, Coats AJS, The increased ventilatory response to exercise in chronic heart failure: relation to pulmonary pathology, Heart 1997; 77: p.138-146.

Davidson JT, Whipp BJ, Wasserman K, Koyal SN, Lugliani R, Role of the carotid bodies in breath-holding, New England Journal of Medicine 1974 April 11; 290(15): p. 819-822.

Denko NC, Fontana LA, Hudson KM, Sutphin PD, Raychaudhuri S, Altman R, Giaccia AJ, Investigating hypoxic tumor physiology through gene expression patterns, Oncogene 2003 September 1; 22(37): p. 5907-5914.

Dimopoulou I, Tsintzas OK, Alivizatos PA, Tzelepis GE, Pattern of breathing during progressive exercise in chronic heart failure, Int J Cardiol. 2001 Dec; 81(2-3): p. 117-121.

Elborn JS, Riley M, Stanford CF, Nicholls DP, The effects of flosequinan on submaximal exercise in patients with chronic cardiac failure, Br J Clin Pharmacol. 1990 May; 29(5): p.519-524.

Epstein SK, Zilberberg MD; Facoby C, Ciubotaru RL, Kaplan LM, Response to symptom-limited exercise in patients with the hepatopulmonary syndrome, Chest 1998; 114; p. 736-741.

Esquivel E, Chaussain M, Plouin P, Ponsot G, Arthuis M, Physical exercise and voluntary hyperventilation in childhood absence epilepsy, Electroencephalogr Clin Neurophysiol 1991 Aug; 79(2): p. 127-132.

Evans SM & Koch CJ, Prognostic significance of tumor oxygenation in humans, Cancer Letters 2003 May 30; 195(1): p. 1-16.

Fanfulla F, Mortara , Maestri R, Pinna GD, Bruschi C, Cobelli F, Rampulla C, The development of hyperventilation in patients with chronic heart failure and Cheyne-Stokes respiration, Chest 1998; 114; p. 1083-1090.

Ford MJ, Camilleri MJ, Hanson RB, Wiste JA, Joyner MJ, Hyperventilation, central autonomic control, and colonic tone in humans, Gut 1995 Oct; 37(4): p. 499-504.

Fried R, Fox MC, Carlton RM, Effect of diaphragmatic respiration with end-tidal CO_2 biofeedback on respiration, EEG, and seizure frequency in idiopathic epilepsy, Annals of New York Academy of Sciences 1990; 602: p. 67-96.

Han JN, Stegen K, Simkens K, Cauberghs M, Schepers R, Van den Bergh O, Clément J, Van de Woestijne KP, Unsteadiness of breathing in patients with hyperventilation syndrome and anxiety disorders, Eur Respir J 1997; 10: p. 167–176.

Harris AL, Hypoxia: a key regulatory factor in tumour growth, National Review in Cancer 2002 January; 2(1): p. 38-47.

Henderson Y, Acapnia and shock. - I. Carbon dioxide as a factor in the regulation of the heart rate, American Journal of Physiology 1908, 21: p. 126- 156.

Johnson BD, Beck KC, Olson LJ, O'Malley KA, Allison TG, Squires RW, Gau GT, Ventilatory constraints during exercise in patients with chronic heart failure, Chest 2000 Feb; 117(2): p. 321-332.

Johnson BD, Scanlon PD, Beck KC, Regulation of ventilatory capacity during exercise in asthmatics, Journal of Applied Physiology 1995 September; 79(3): p. 892-901.

Breathing Slower and Less: The Greatest Health Discovery Ever

Kahaly GJ, Nieswandt J, Wagner S, Schlegel J, Mohr-Kahaly S, Hommel G, Ineffective cardiorespiratory function in hyperthyroidism, Journal of Clinical Endocrinology and Metabolism 1998 November; 83(11): p. 4075-4078.

Kassabian J, Miller KD, Lavietes MH, Respiratory center output and ventilatory timing in patients with acute airway (asthma) and alveolar (pneumonia) disease, Chest 1982 May; 81(5): p.536-543.

Kohn RM & Cutcher B, Breath-holding time in the screening for rehabilitation potential of cardiac patients, Scandinavian Journal of Rehabilitation Medicine 1970; 2(2): p. 105-107.

Kunz M & Ibrahim SM, Molecular responses to hypoxia in tumor cells, Molecular Cancer 2003; 2: p. 23-31.

MacKinnon DF, Craighead B, Hoehn-Saric R, Carbon dioxide provocation of anxiety and respiratory response in bipolar disorder, J Affect Disord 2007 Apr; 99(1-3): p.45-49.

Mancini M, Filippelli M, Seghieri G, Iandelli I, Innocenti F, Duranti R, Scano G, Respiratory Muscle Function and Hypoxic Ventilatory Control in Patients With Type I Diabetes, Chest 1999; 115; p.1553-1562.

McFadden ER & Lyons HA, Arterial-blood gases in asthma, The New England Journal of Medicine 1968 May 9, 278 (19): p. 1027-1032.

Mora JD, Grant L, Kenyon P, Patel MK, Jenner FA, Respiratory ventilation and carbon dioxide levels in syndromes of depression, Br J Psychiatry 1976 Nov, 129: p. 457-464.

Newton E, Hyperventilation Syndrome 2004 June 17, Topic 270, p. 1-7 (www.emedicine.com).

Pain MC, Biddle N, Tiller JW, Panic disorder, the ventilatory response to carbon dioxide and respiratory variables, Psychosom Med 1988 Sep-Oct; 50(5): p. 541-548.

Palange P, Valli G, Onorati P, Antonucci R, Paoletti P, Rosato A, Manfredi F, Serra P, Effect of heliox on lung dynamic hyperinflation, dyspnea, and exercise endurance capacity in COPD patients, J Appl Physiol. 2004 Nov; 97(5): p.1637-1642.

Perez-Padilla R, Cervantes D, Chapela R, Selman M, Rating of breathlessness at rest during acute asthma: correlation with spirometry and usefulness of breath-holding time, Revistade Investigacion Clinica 1989 July-September; 41(3): p. 209-213.

Physiology, Fourth edition, ed. by Berne, Robert M. & Levy Matthew N.; Mosby, St.Louis, 1998.

Radwan L, Maszczyk Z, Koziorowski A, Koziej M, Cieslicki J, Sliwinski P, Zielinski J, Control of breathing in obstructive sleep apnoea and in patients with the overlap syndrome, Eur Respir J. 1995 Apr; 8(4): p.542-545.

Rockwell S, Oxygen delivery: implications for the biology and therapy of solid tumors, Oncology Research 1997; 9(6-7): p. 383-390.

Ryan H, Lo J, Johnson RS, The hypoxia inducible factor-1 gene is required for embryogenesis and solid tumor formation, EMBO Journal 1998, 17: p. 3005- 3015.

Ryan HE, Poloni M, McNulty W, Elson D, Gassmann M, Arbeit JM, Johnson RS, Hypoxia-inducible factor-1 is a positive factor in solid tumor growth, Cancer Res, August 1, 2000; 60(15): p. 4010 - 4015.

Schmaltz C, Hardenbergh PH, Wells A, Fisher DE, Regulation of proliferationsurvival decisions during tumor cell hypoxia, Molecular and Cellular Biology 1998 May, 18(5): p. 2845-2854.

Sinderby C, Spahija J, Beck J, Kaminski D, Yan S, Comtois N, Sliwinski P, Diaphragm activation during exercise in chronic obstructive pulmonary disease, Am J Respir Crit Care Med 2001 Jun; 163(7): 1637-1641.

Sterling GM, The mechanism of bronchoconstriction due to hypocapnia in man, Clinical Science 1968 April; 34(2): p. 277-285.

Stulbarg MS, Winn WR, Kellett LE, Bilateral Carotid Body Resection for the Relief of Dyspnea in Severe Chronic Obstructive Pulmonary Disease, Chest 1989; 95 (5): p.1123-1128.

Tantucci C, Bottini P, Dottorini ML, Puxeddu E, Casucci G, Scionti L, Sorbini CA, Ventilatory response to exercise in diabetic subjects with autonomic neuropathy, J Appl Physiol 1996, 81(5): p.1978–1986.

Tantucci C, Bottini P, Fiorani C, Dottorini ML, Santeusanio F, Provinciali L, Sorbini CA, Casucci G, Cerebrovascular reactivity and hypercapnic respiratory drive in diabetic autonomic neuropathy, J Appl Physiol 2001, 90: p. 889–896.

Tantucci C, Scionti L, Bottini P, Dottorini ML, Puxeddu E, Casucci G, Sorbini CA, Influence of autonomic neuropathy of different severities on the hypercapnic drive to breathing in diabetic patients, Chest. 1997 Jul; 112(1): p. 145-153.

Tepper RS, Skatrud B, Dempsey JA, Ventilation and oxygenation changes during sleep in cystic fibrosis, Chest 1983; 84; p. 388-393.

Travers J, Dudgeon DJ, Amjadi K, McBride I, Dillon K, Laveneziana P, Ofir D, Webb KA, O'Donnell DE, Mechanisms of exertional dyspnea in patients with cancer, J Appl Physiol 2008 Jan; 104(1): p.57-66.

Chapter 4. Breathing and quality of life

Introduction

What does it mean, "to be sick"? Medical professionals would tell you that being sick means being diagnosed with a certain disease. However, for the average person being sick implies an inability to lead a normal life. This includes many factors, such as emotional well-being, good relationships with others, doing one's job well, sound and refreshing sleep, joy of physical activity, good appetite, effective digestion, and many other elements of our minds and bodies. All these factors can be included under the heading, "quality of life".

When we are sick, usually all these parameters are affected. Jobs are done poorly, emotional problems or depression are normal, one's mood is unstable, ordinary events can be annoying, usual conversations can be irritable, relationships with others suffer, sleep is longer and less refreshing, physical work is hard, appetite is weak, digestion is sluggish, etc. Why does all this happen at the same time? Now we know that breathing gets heavier with the progression of a disease. Can breathing and its effects provide the answer to this question? Indeed, since breathing influences every cell, tissue, organ and system of the human organism, it can also influence the "quality of life" factors we discussed above. Let us consider some of these connections using explanations based on known CO_2 effects.

4.1 Can heavy breathing cause problems with sleep?

Why do we need sleep? Our understanding of sleep is very limited and incomplete. Common sense tells us that we need it to provide rest for the brain and muscles. We know that deep breathing makes the brain over-excited and muscles tense. Hence, CO_2 deficiency can affect the quality of our sleep due to these effects. Here are some general practical observations about breathing and the quality of sleep.

Breathing Slower and Less: The Greatest Health Discovery Ever
A person with normal breathing (about 60 s CP):

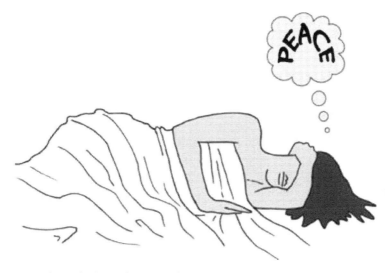

- falls asleep in less than 1 minute;
- sleeps for about 4-5 hours and it can stay in the same position the whole night;
- does not remember dreams and does not have nightmares;
- awakes feeling refreshed and full of energy and vigor with a morning CP of about 60 or more seconds.

When the CP is about 15-25 s (as is common for people today), a person:
- may need more time to fall asleep (up to 5-30 minutes or more);
- can sleep up to 7-9 hours and in different positions;
- can remember dreams and may have nightmares;
- wakes up feeling tired, often with about 10 seconds CP due to morning hyperventilation.

Why? During the previous day and night, this individual has had chronically low tissue O2 and CO2 stores. The muscles were tense, instead of naturally relaxed, and the brain hypoxic and over-excited, instead of calm. Even during sleep, the brain, due to hyperventilation, remained abnormally excited (remember "spontaneous and asynchronous firing of cortical neurons"?) and hypoxic.

Consider severely sick, terminally ill or hospitalized patients with a typical CP of about 5-10 s or even less.

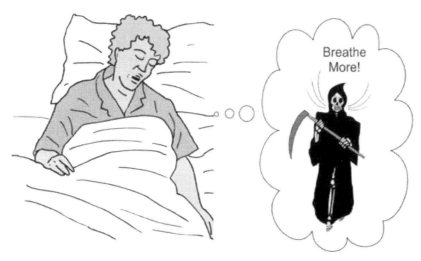

These people:
- may need even more time to fall asleep (up to 30 minutes or more);

- can sleep up to 12-15 hours tossing and turning in bed;
- can remember many dreams and often have nightmares;
- awaken feeling tired and sluggish.

Their quality of sleep is often miserable. Why? Because these people, due to severe chronic hyperventilation, have critically low oxygenation and CO_2 values. They are chronically very tense and over-excited. Their muscles and brain need much more time to rest and relax. However, this is difficult or impossible, since O_2 and CO_2 stores are critically low, during the night as well.

Some people (Professor Buteyko, some Russian Buteyko doctors, Western Buteyko practitioners and students, and hatha yoga masters) have/had very light breathing (about 3 l/min for ventilation) with 2-3 minutes CP. Such people need only about 2 hours of sleep during the night. Why? High CO2 concentrations keep the muscles relaxed and the brain calm throughout the day and night. Normally these people do not need much sleep at all, since they are resting even while they work!

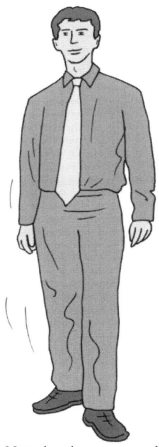

Note that there are people who may have only 5-10 s CP and have no problems or complaints about sleep.

Occasionally, some people may have 30-35 s CP and still be concerned or unhappy about their quality of sleep.

However, all these cases are exceptions rather than the rule. It can be of important practical and scientific value to find out the exact biochemical, neurological and psychological links between breathing and quality of sleep

Why do most people have problems with sleep when they breathe more? Why some people are less affected?

Be observant. If you know the CPs of your friends and relatives, investigate, if possible, whether this general correlation between the CP and quality of sleep is correct for them. Also, check, if it works for you on different days (your CP and sleep quality can vary from day to day due to diseases, infections, exercise, stress, etc.).

Warning. Remember that CP measurements are done until the first desire to breathe. Your health and quality of sleep would not be better if you push yourself to get higher numbers. In fact, if you later gasp for air, your breathing can become even worse. It is how you breathe twenty-four hours a day, seven days a week that matter.

Questions. Who would survive longer in the jungle or wild forests, or in other natural conditions: those who have 15-20 s second CPs and need to sleep up to 7-9 hours (with tossing, snoring, wheezing, panting) or those with 2-3 min CP, who need only 2 hours of noiseless sleep in the same body position? (Note that conditions in the wild normally imply the presence of ever hungry predators.) What were the CPs of primitive people? What can be said about their health, and their physical and psychological well-being? Is there a case for saying that primitive people did not suffer from many modern diseases?

4.2 Are breathing and digestion connected?

Hyperventilation is an important part of our "fight-or-flight" response. In such conditions, large muscles need more blood for a better chance of survival. That means that more blood would be diverted to the large skeletal muscles, resulting in less blood for vital organs, including the organs of digestion. Indeed, British and Japanese scientists found decreased blood flow to the liver (Hughes et al, 1979 and Okazaki et al, 1980), while American medical doctors confirmed the same effect for the colon (Gilmour et al, 1980). Hence, the more heavily we breathe, the less blood goes to our digestive organs.

In addition, the suppressed Bohr effect reduces oxygenation of the digestive organs, as documented by various Western studies.

Almost a century ago, Yale Professor Yandell Henderson from Yale's School of Medicine found that a low CO_2 in the arterial blood (due to hyperventilation) resulted in loss of tone of the intestines, producing extreme intestinal congestion.

Saturation of the blood with CO_2 rapidly eliminated the congestion (Henderson, 1907). The results were published in the American Journal of Physiology.

Warning. In some people, mild voluntary hyperventilation can almost halt their digestion so that it can take up to 5-7 or more hours to empty the stomach. Note that such "experimentation" can be dangerous leading to the aggravation of existing gastrointestinal problems. Breathing less (or hypoventilation) can also make some digestive problems worse.

Hence, chronic hyperventilation can interfere with normal digestion. Poor blood and oxygen supply can lead to a lack of digestive enzymes, accumulation of metabolic waste products, slower digestion, putrefaction of some foods and nutrients and mal-absorption. Systematic research in this area is absent and there are more questions than answers.

From a practical viewpoint, the above suggests that smaller CPs correspond to slower digestion. For example, a person with about a 60 s CP may need about 1- 1.5 hours to digest a regular meal (when almost no food is left in the stomach). The same meal for a sick individual (e.g., 10-15 s CP) would need 1-2 more hours of digestion. The person with normal breathing after this meal would still be reasonably fit and able to exercise (not very rigorously, of course) after eating the same meal. The sick person would definitely need a rest.

Be observant. When we are acutely sick with the flue, cold or other infection or disease, our CP probably decreases about 2 or more times from its usual level. What happens with your digestion? How would you feel if you were to eat your regular meal while sick? What would happen with your CP? Which meals and foods do you prefer when you are sick?

Questions. For primitive people, it was vital to defend themselves any time, day and night, including after meals. Could they be physically strong and mentally fit after meals if their usual CPs were about 20-25 s (as in a modern population)? What would you expect their usual CPs to be?

4.3 What is the link between breathing and common body postures?

People with normal breathing prefer to spend their days standing even when there are chairs, armchairs, sofas and couches available. According to Professor Buteyko, being upright is the most natural body position; this was the norm during almost the entire history of humanity. Standing also was the norm in factories, plants, shops and offices up to the beginning of the 20th century.

Standing, while maintaining a straight spine, allows the diaphragm and other organs below it to be freely suspended. The diaphragm is easily movable and can be relaxed. Breathing naturally becomes light. CO_2 concentrations in healthy people become higher in comparison with other body postures.

Most modern people (with 15-25 s CP) prefer to sit, since their muscles, due to a moderate hypoxia and CO_2 deficiency, are too tense for prolonged standing. Moreover, excessive tension in the shoulders, neck and chest muscles often causes slouching while sitting and often when standing. The gait of modern people also shows signs of stress and muscular tension.

Sick people (e.g., 5-10 s CP) like to lie down during the day as well as at night. Chronic fatigue (see the next section) is a common complaint. Severely ill patients often lie for days and nights, since even sitting requires their muscular and mental efforts.

(Traditional hatha yoga teaching suggests that hatha yoga masters can hold their breath for 3-5 minutes. Old manuscripts in hatha yoga mentioned that such people could freely move in space and possibly fly!?)

4.4 How is the joy of physical activity related to breathing?

Large CPs also mean that all tissues, including the muscles, have normal and sufficient amounts of oxygen and the body is full of energy. Indeed, a person with an over 60 s CP can walk 2-3 floors upstairs while holding his/her breath and can resume light nasal breathing at the top. It is difficult to imagine that physical activity is hard for him/her.

Normal breathing means enjoyment of physical activity. It is not a problem for a person with over 60 s CP to be physically active for 8, 10 or 12 hours. Activities can include walking, gardening, or doing various jobs around the house every day without feeling tired. Such a person would be happy and willing to do some physical activity or job at any part of the day.

When we have 15-25 s CP frequent or constant complaints about feeling tired and lack of energy are normal. The brain, due to abnormal excitement, can get "creative" and it can easily invent "reasons" and "theories" why certain errands or jobs are undesirable or not possible. Coffee, chocolate, and sugar are among the substances frequently used to boost energy levels. Without such stimulants, it can be hard and stressful to force oneself to do work.

Are there any medical studies? A group of British doctors from the Department of Cardiology in Charing Cross Hospital, London tested 100 consecutive patients diagnosed with chronic fatigue syndrome, according to their article in the Journal of Royal Society of Medicine (Rosen et al, 1990). Ninety-three patients had chronic hyperventilation. If the doctors had used a stricter definition of hyperventilation (less than 40 mm Hg CO2 in blood), probably all 100 people would have been diagnosed with chronic hyperventilation.

When the CP is critically low (e.g., less than 10 s), chronic fatigue is a typical experience for most people. Hospitalized and severely sick patients usually have low CPs. They have very little, if any, desire to exercise (even lightly) or walk.

Indeed, physical effort could cause acute episodes and severe problems with their health.

When their CPs are low (10-20 seconds), most people are going to complain that they are tired. Some individuals can be mentally excited and physically active, while others, especially children, may be restless and hyperactive (e.g., with Attention Deficit Hyperactivity Disorder). That happens because of our individual responses to deep breathing.

With 20-30 seconds for the current CP, most people can do moderate or even quite intensive physical exercise with nose breathing only. Nose breathing is the crucial factor that makes exercise safe and very effective to increase body O2 content. Exercise becomes much easier and more pleasant. It is not a burden anymore.

With 30-40 s for the morning CP, exercise is very easy. Nose breathing requires little efforts.

However, the true benefits of breathing retraining comes with 40-60+ s for the morning CP when people start to really enjoy and, in most cases, crave physical exercise. Here is the summary of findings.

Body-oxygen level	Desire or abilities to exercise
1-5 s CP	Any physical activity can be life-threatening since acute exacerbation can occur due to the severe degree of overbreathing and critically low body oxygen level.
5-10 s CP	Any exercise, even slow walking on the flat surface, is hard due to severe dyspnea. It can cause exacerbation of health problems (asthma attacks, angina, seizures, and so forth).
11-20 s CP	Most people experience and complain about chronic fatigue, but can walk with only nose breathing for hours on a flat surface.
20-30 s CP	There are few or no complaints about fatigue. Physical activity (e.g., easy relaxed jogging) is well tolerated, but requires considerable psychological effort and self-discipline.
30-40 s CP	Exercise is pleasant and relatively easy, but a systematic or daily exercise routine generally requires good self-discipline.
40-60 s daily CP, less than 40 s morning CP	Exercise is easy and pleasant, nose breathing during exercise is natural and comfortable
Over 40 morning CP	Exercise is a joy and people are full of energy provided that they have enough food to eat. They crave exercise naturally. If they force themselves not to exercise, their CP drops.

4.5 Which feelings and emotions can people experience because of hyperventilation?

Studies found that people become duller and less able to concentrate because of chronic over-breathing. In addition, because of "spontaneous and asynchronous firing of cortical neurons", people can become impulsive, moody, inconsistent, anxious, irritated, intolerant, disrespectful, depressed, hyperactive, verbally abusive, jealous, envious, greedy, and addicted to various unnatural substances and activities. During over-breathing, it becomes more and more difficult to control irrational emotions. Confusion is another common result of over-breathing.

(Note that normal breathing does not guarantee a complete absence of irrational emotions. Upbringing and environmental factors are also important. However, for most people, destructive or self-defeating behavior is possible or more likely in conditions of hyperventilation.)

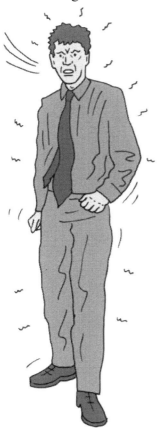

Due to tense muscles, CO_2 deficient people can easily become poorly coordinated, over-active, aggressive, or even violent (see right). This often leads to destructive behavior, which requires self-justification on the part of the perpetrators. How is that possible? Physiology has proved that the nerve cells become irritable during hyperventilation. As a result, the brain, instead of being a tool for the exploration of the world and the analysis of one's own behavior, often becomes a tool for the invention of excuses.

Be observant. Watching TV for example, what can you (always?) say about the breathing of people who are violent or angry? Have you ever seen people expressing violent or angry behavior while having normal or invisible breathing?

4.6 Which personal skills and abilities are affected?

In a state of chronic hyperventilation, various professional, technical, perceptual, peacemaking, psychological, athletic, recreational and other abilities and skills deteriorate. These include: concentration, short- and long-term memory, logical and analytical abilities, the work of all the senses, coordination, precision of movements, balance, abilities to negotiate, to compromise, to be consistent, persistent, disciplined, self-organized, etc.

4.7 What about the influence of temporary hyperventilation on performance?

Physiological studies have shown inconsistent results. Even within the same study, individual results under the same conditions can be different. Some people can perform reasonably well, some not. Why? Abnormal excitement causes two effects. On the one hand, highways of communication in our electrical brains get more "ready". On the other hand, there is more interference from irrelevant sources.

That can explain why reaction time, memory, and logical skills can be sometimes improved by breathing more. At other times or for other people, they become worse. Why then are the overall effects of chronic hyperventilation negative? Experience shows that it affects our attitudes, feelings and emotions in the destructive ways discussed above.

4.8 What is the impact of breathing on perception of the outer world?

Normal perception requires a calm brain so that our senses and nerve cells can freely transmit correct information for objective analysis. In other words, we need minimal abnormal interference from our nervous system (self-generated signals) during the process of communication and analysis.

Hyperventilation, on the other hand, plays a key role in our immediate reaction to stress or in an emergency situation when our well-being or life is in danger. At such moments we do not need the objective world. We need to save/fight for our lives. Hence our minds need threats, enemies, stress sources or outside problems to deal with.

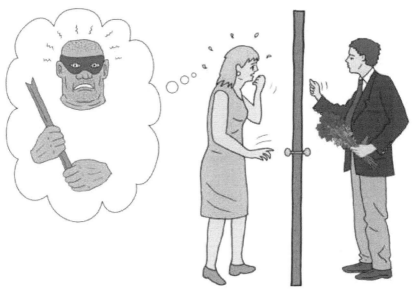

Sometimes an obvious or visible threat is absent (no enemies or threats are seen). Then the excited brain can invent threats literally from nothing due to "spontaneous and asynchronous ...". Hence, when we breathe more, we have a tendency to unconsciously search for threats, enemies, problems, etc.

4.9 How can people react when there is a lack of normal perception?

There is only one real world, but a person sees it differently at different moments in time. That usually means that people also see their own positions and places in this world differently. Some people experience mood swings. Sometimes, they can feel helpless and weak; sometimes they can feel themselves powerful and invincible.

In such conditions they are likely to deny one state while being in another. Realization and acceptance/self-analysis of these changes can lead to periods of depression and confusion. Addictions can develop as ways to avoid this abnormal perception.

4.10 How are addictions connected to breathing?

The practice of Russian medical doctors revealed that addictions (to street drugs, sugar, coffee, smoking, alcohol, etc.) among patients with deep breathing (when the CP are below 15-20 s) are fairly common. Few people were able to quit addictions to, for example, sugar, coffee, and smoking even when professional help was offered based on persuasion and appeals to reason.

When one's CP increases to 35-40 s these addictions usually disappear. In other words, addictions and normal breathing have a hard time coexisting together. Imagine that a person is now full of energy and vigor all the time. His/her senses and perception function normally. Would he/she need drugs, sugar, coffee or many other substances or unnatural activities?

Many street drugs (e.g., cocaine and marijuana) suppress breathing. Medical studies show that they can temporarily increase breath holding abilities 3-4 times.

Under such conditions, the nervous system functions much better. Sounds are richer, colors are brighter, smells are stronger. The addict becomes smarter, better coordinated and more confident. "Feeling high" is an expression used for these times. Sudden transition from hyperventilation to normal breathing is probably one of the main causes of this effect. When healthy people quickly recover from severe diseases (e.g., overnight), they can experience similar changes and feelings.

4.11 Can being overweight be caused by hyperventilation?

We already discussed weight gain in the previous chapter. Here are more details.

Hyperventilation interferes with normal weight in different ways:

1. It makes people lazy and less able to exercise.

2. Many people have a tendency to snack or overeat in order to cope with stress or depression.

3. Hyperventilation makes regulation of blood sugar abnormal due to changes in the concentrations and production of certain hormones (e.g., insulin, glycogen, and cortisol).

4. CO_2 deficiency, according to limited Russian research, changes the permeability of cellular membranes in relation to glucose and other substances. More blood glucose can be driven into fat cells.

5. Experience shows that hyperventilation changes tastes and food preferences of people so that they become addicted to junk foods.

Most people react to heavier breathing by poorer blood glucose control, being hungrier, eating more, exercising less and gradually gaining extra weight.

As I have seen in all my overweight students, when they start to slow down their breathing and increase their CP, they report less hunger for foods, more energy and fast weight loss.

4.12 Is there a connection between taking medication and breathing?

When the CP is 60 or more seconds, such people do not need medication.

Moreover, as it was mentioned above in relation to addictions, healthy people feel comfortable and perform well without use of street drugs, sugar, coffee, tobacco, and other unnatural substances.

When the CP is below 35-40 s, the amount or dosage often varies, in relation to the difference, proportionally. For example, a patient with 10 s CP would need about twice as much medication than the same patient with 20 s CP in order to have similar symptom-reduction effects.

Drugs prescribed by a doctor usually address certain symptoms the patient is complaining about. Often these drugs suppress the symptom(s) and the patient can feel better for a while. However, symptoms are just expressions of some pathological processes. But drugs do not address the fundamental causes of the disease.

It is normal then that the body remains sick or gets even sicker. Hence, other symptoms get worse, while the old symptoms need more medication due to physiological habituation.

Symptoms show us that something is wrong and some measures must be taken. Drugs, therefore, create an illusion that the pathology is corrected, but the body will likely protest even more.

Indeed, most medical drugs intensify respiration since they are foreign for the human body and are to be eliminated by various organs (kidneys, liver, skin, etc.).

Another big problem relates to the dosage of medication chosen by the doctor. This problem can be difficult since the degree of symptoms does not always correspond to the visible severity of the disease.

Some drugs, especially hormones, can be useful or even necessary in order to assist recovery of normal breathing in certain situations. The CP is the main measuring tool of the progress achieved and the required dosages.

Decades of professional medical research in Russia, and now in other countries, show that gradual normalization of breathing allows gradual elimination of medication. In relation to asthma, these medication-reduction guidelines in relation to hormones can be found in the book Living without asthma: the Buteyko method (Novozhilov, 2004) written by Andrey Novozhilov, MD, chief doctor of the Moscow Buteyko Clinic.

4.13 Does over-breathing make life less meaningful?

A meaningful life means, among many other things, an ability to be realistic, the absence of addictions, having good and healthy relationships with others, the abilities to work productively, to enjoy physical work, to achieve certain goals in life, etc. Let us consider those dimensions, which are not discussed above.

Meaningful relationships with others are possible when the person has a long- term caring and respectful attitude towards others. He/she can clearly see:
- one's own and others' abilities and limitations (who is who);
- how they can help each other;
- the impact of relationships on both sides;
- the dynamic or future trends in interactions.

Seeing these things clearly is more difficult in an abnormal mental state.

Hyperventilating people are more likely to be inconsistent (or moody), choose the wrong friends, pay attention to wrong or non-existent problems in their relationships with other people, etc.

4.14 Do we accomplish less in a personal life when breathing is heavy?

The achievement of personal goals (e.g., in business and employment, personal life and hobbies, arts and sports) requires:
- an ability to perceive reality normally and to be objective when considering one's skills, growth potentials and limitations;
- an ability to choose an optimum plan to achieve the selected goals;
- an ability to work diligently and persistently towards these goals day after day, month after month, and often year after year while

being under the influence of different outer and inner destabilizing factors and processes.

Chronic over-breathing negatively affects the whole goal-achieving complex. An objective perception of the real world, including one's own place and qualities, is more difficult or nearly impossible. Choosing the optimum plan for actions and its execution become problematic. (If one cannot see oneself clearly, how can one make a good plan?). Finally, an inconsistent state of mind ("spontaneous and asynchronous …") makes self-discipline, diligence and persistence, in relation to daily work for many days/months/years, impossible or too difficult.

4.15 What problems in society would be solved if normal breathing were again, as long time ago, a norm of life for most people?

During the 1910's the commanding officers of British Air Force personnel used breath-holding time as a test for pilots. When the pilots failed the test, they were barred from flying planes. It was expected that after full exhalation and a usual inhale, a pilot should be able to keep his breath for at least 50 s (That corresponds to about a 35 s CP). Military medical doctor Lieutenant-Colonel Martin Flack conducted thousands of such measurements. The results of these studies were described in his article Some simple tests of physical efficiency published in one of the most respected medical magazines, The Lancet in 1919 (Flack, 1919). Why was the test important? They found that pilots with short breath holding time could crash their planes and kill themselves due to stress.

Since modern people have on average a 20-30 s CP, should we be surprised by our performance in many areas, from families to states? In my view, the high rates of personal conflicts, lawsuits, divorces, number of children growing in broken families, rates of numerous mental disorders, addictions, international conflicts and wars, and many other similar phenomena and effects could be reduced 5-10 times or more or completely eliminated, if everybody has normal breathing. Obviously, these claims need more scientific and clinical research.

Many historians, religious persons, politicians, psychologists, philosophers and humanists have been concerned about the variety of social problems that have appeared during the last 100 years due to fear. Fear, as it was acknowledged, has been a nightmare for humanity. It has expressed itself in the destructive tendencies found in various social units (families, communities, countries, societies, etc.). Fear is another by-product of hyperventilation.

Note that the breathing characteristics of ordinary people during previous centuries were better than those of the upper classes, including political, social, military, economical, and other leaders. Indeed, upper class people and leaders have always been affected by less exercise, more sitting, abnormal changes in diet especially due to overeating and cooked and processed foods, overheating, more speaking and other activities and conditions considered unnatural for a human being. The influence of these factors on breathing will be discussed in the next chapter.

In my view, normal breathing and over 60 s CP should be a requirement in a healthy society to take/have any state or official job. This would apply for all political, social, security, military, health, educational and other leaders and managers, as well as ordinary people.

References for Chapter 4

Flack M, Some simple tests of physical efficiency, Lancet 1920; 196: p. 210-212.

Gilmour DG, Douglas IH, Aitkenhead AR, Hothersall AP, Horton PW, Ledingham IM, Colon blood flow in the dog: effects of changes in arterial carbon dioxide tension, Cardiovascular Research 1980 Jan; 14(1): p. 11-20.

Henderson Y, Production of shock by loss of carbon dioxide, and relief by partial asphyxiation, American Journal of Physiology 1907, 19: p. XIV-XV.

Hughes RL, Mathie RT, Fitch W, Campbell D, Liver blood flow and oxygen consumption during hypocapnia and IPPV in the greyhound, Journal of Applied Physiology 1979 Aug; 47(2): p. 290-295.

Novozhilov A, Living without asthma: the Buteyko method, 2nd edition, Mobiwell Verlag, Frildberg, Germany, 2004.

Okazaki K, Hashimoto K, Okutsu Y, Okumura F, Effect of arterial carbon dioxide tension on regional myocardial tissue oxygen tension in the dog [Article in Japanese], Masui 1991 Nov; 40(11): p. 1620-1624.

Okazaki K, Okutsu Y, Fukunaga A, Effect of carbon dioxide (hypocapnia and hypercapnia) on tissue blood flow and oxygenation of liver, kidneys and skeletal muscle in the dog [Article in Japanese], Masui 1989 Apr, 38 (4): p. 457-464.

Rosen SD, King JC, Wilkinson JB, Nixon PG, Is chronic fatigue syndrome synonymous with effort syndrome? Journal of Royal Society of Medicine 1990 Dec; 83(12): p. 761-764.

Chapter 5. Why do we breathe too heavily?

Introduction

Western physiological norms for breathing were established about 100 years ago.

Typical CO_2 concentrations in the lungs and arterial blood were about 5.5-6%, with a lung ventilation of about 5-6 l/min. The usual CPs of ordinary people were in a range from 40 to 50 s. The CPs of people nowadays are about 25-30 s. We breathe more air and have lower CO_2 concentrations. We also have less oxygen in our vital organs. Why? Modern civilization and its materialistic values have brought about various changes affecting our breathing and health. The parameters that reduce oxygenation and the CP were shortly discussed in Chapter 1. Let us look at them again in more detail.

5.1 Does an open mouth affect health?

One can observe that modern man often has his/her mouth open (while sitting, standing, reading, working, walking, exercising, etc.). Breathing through one's mouth reduces CO_2 levels in the lungs and, hence, in the whole body. Why? Nasal breathing creates more resistance to airflow. Hence, we can tolerate higher CO_2 concentrations in the lungs and blood since more work to ventilate the lungs is required to keep the same CO_2 levels during nasal breathing. The difference is especially large during physical exercise. In addition, mouth breathing makes the volume of the dead space smaller. (The dead space is the air reservoir between the lungs and outer air.) This intermediate reservoir helps us to have higher CO_2 concentrations in the lungs.

Finally, nasal passages produce nitric oxide (NO), a gas that is to be inhaled into the lungs and absorbed in the blood for dilation of blood vessels. Many heart patients use nitroglycerine and some other heart drugs, which release nitric oxide into the bloodstream. However, heart patients often breathe through the mouth; thereby, losing their own best source for NO which is produced naturally by the body.

Similarly, when the nose becomes blocked, people open their mouths for breathing. This makes their problem worse. The nose can get completely blocked due to constriction of small blood vessels and reduced blood supply.

Was the situation in relation to mouth breathing different in the past? In order to detect historical changes, you can investigate photos and movies made, for example, 30 or more years ago. Was it normal, then, for people to have open mouths for breathing?

5.2 Is physical inactivity a factor?

Our primitive ancestors were physically active for 6-12 hours every day.

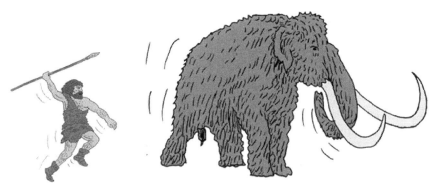

We, on average, are active for about 1-2 hours per day or often less. Too little physical exercise depresses metabolism and oxygen transport, gradually causing chronic hyperventilation. Russian practical observations revealed that, if a healthy individual (with about 60 s CP) has only 1-2 hours or less of daily physical activity, his/her breathing will be getting worse and worse. The CP can drop down to about 30-35 s or even less.

Note that even during physical exercise we should keep our mouths closed. Unfortunately, it is rare to meet a person who exercises with his/her mouth closed all the time.

How healthy should we be in order to exercise? Practical experience of Soviet and Russian doctors revealed that exercise is inadvisable for people with low CPs (below about 20 s). Physical exercise does not provide maximum benefits when people breathe through their mouths while exercising. In these cases CO2 stores usually get smaller. Breathing and the CP can get worse for many hours after such an exercise. When the CP is critically low (as with severely sick people), exercise becomes dangerous.

5.3 What about overeating?

The digestive system is a sophisticated conveyor more complicated than any modern chemical factory. It has its own brain (the enteric nervous system), various organs, special chemical messengers for communication, and dozens of digestive enzymes. When we are hungry, the system is ready to accept and process food. Eating without real hunger results in biochemical stress for some organs and the whole system in general. (According to recent surveys, over 60% of American women eat or have a snack when they feel stressed.) Stress, in its turn, leads to hyperventilation.

5.4 What breathing changes occur during sleep?

During sleep, as each hour passes, breathing gets deeper and heavier for most people. That is easy to check using the CP. The CP drop is especially noticeable after 4-6 hours of sleep. (We are physiologically created to sleep less than 4-5 hours.)

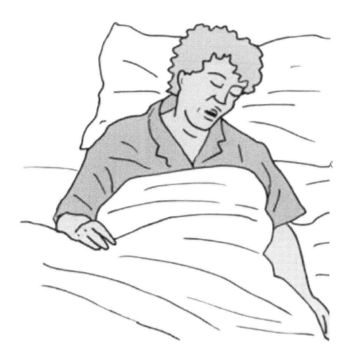

Russian studies also revealed that different sleeping positions have different effects on breathing. Sleeping on one's back is worst. It is one of the main causes of poor health for many modern people. CO_2 losses at night are particularly high when people breathe through open mouth while sleeping on the back.

Practice shows that sleeping on the left side or on the stomach (or chest) is optimal for most people.

5.5 Can overheating make us breathe more?

Our clothes, homes, offices, and other building are often too warm. At the same time, our inner body temperature should be kept in a very narrow range (about 36-37° C when we are healthy). Usually body heat is removed through the skin.

If that is not possible, the only way to get rid of extra heat is by overbreathing.

When the weather gets cold, we wear warmer clothes. However, most people continue to wear over-warm clothing in transport, shopping centers, stores, and other public areas or buildings.

Question. When overheated, people feel that something is not right with their system. Indeed, overheating can cause asthma and heart attacks, migraine headaches, stroke and other unpleasant effects. How can overheating lead to these problems?

5.6 What about poor posture and tense muscles?

Poor posture results in stress and tension in various muscles. Tense muscles distort our natural grace and elegance. That is a normal response to hyperventilation. Tense muscles help us to prepare for physical activity during the fight-or-flight response.

Many modern people have muscular tension, especially in the neck-jaws-shoulders-chest muscles. That usually results in slouching, especially while sitting.

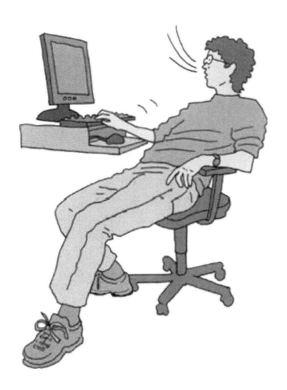

Why is slouching unhealthy? Consider a person with normal breathing (60 s CP) who starts sitting in a slouching position. The diaphragm becomes compressed and almost immobile. Normal diaphragmatic breathing is impossible and chest muscles get involved in the breathing process. However, this chest breathing is deeper (usually by about 50-80%) than previous diaphragmatic breathing and the CP of a healthy person is likely to drop down to at least 30-35 s.

Sick people also experience similar effects. They have deeper breathing and shorter CPs when they slouch. Normal breathing requires that we have a straight spine during all daily activities.

5.7 Do we breathe more while talking?

Breathing Slower and Less: The Greatest Health Discovery Ever

Healthy people, as one Western study found, breathe twice as much air when they speak. That reduces their CO2 stores. Long conversations can thereby lead to dizziness, light-headedness, loss of concentration, emotional instability, muscular tension, abnormal posture and other negative effects.

Moreover, taking deep inhalations, or speaking with loud voice and/or high pitch, or strong emotions, all make breathing heavier.

Questions. What can you say about breathing, emotions, and postures of these talking women? Is this picture typical for modern times?

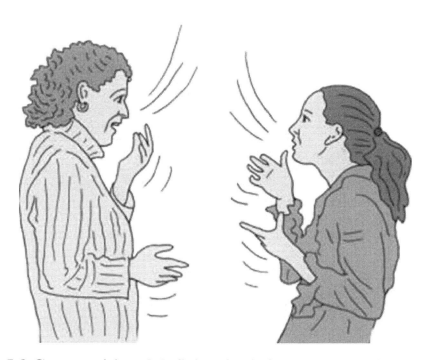

5.8 Can nutritional deficiencies influence breathing?

Due to intensive farming and food refining methods, our food is less nutritious than 100 or more years ago. We get less essential fatty acids (omega oils), calcium/magnesium, fiber, zinc, trace-metals and other essential nutrients.

Nutritional deficiencies, depending on one's personal make-up, create stress for certain organs, body parts, and systems of the human organism. This stress intensifies chronic hyperventilation.

5.9 Can toxic chemicals and pollutants from air, water, food and other sources lead to hyperventilation?

Many industrial chemicals are harmful for the body. For example, pesticides, herbicides, petroleum products, preservatives, colors, heavy metals, and many others can be accumulated in various organs and body parts. These chemicals stress the immune system and organs of elimination. Biochemical stress is also a state of emergency for the human body. This stress also results in hyperventilation.

5.10 Are there any special factors for babies?

Before the baby is born, the fetus gets all its blood supply from the mother through the umbilical cord. This includes CO_2 and O_2. Because of this, the breathing of the fetus depends solely on the mother's breathing and when she hyperventilates, her unborn baby also hyperventilates.

Birth is a severe shock for the baby. Probably, the central part of this shock is a drastic drop (about 30%) in blood CO_2 concentrations. New environmental conditions cause stress and make their breathing heavy. In order to make the transition to new air more gradual, most (maybe all?) primitive and recent cultures used swaddling (or tight wrapping) of babies. That prevented unduly deep chest breathing and restricted their total ventilation. In other words, they breathed less. Modern western civilization and our health care systems have gradually lost this wise cultural tradition.

Warning. Be aware that babies, especially swaddled ones, need normal heat exchange! Excessive clothes can damage their health. Why? Metabolism and heat generation of children is up to 3-4 times more than that for adults. It is too cold for them when their feet or arms are cold. A quick touch by hand can check if the baby is warm or cold. Overheating is one of the leading causes of poor health in modern babies and children.

5.11 Is psychological stress important?

When, how and why do we get stressed psychologically? What are the roots of our maladjusted perception when other people are seen as intrinsically evil?

There are probably very few people on Earth now who have never suffered due to injustice or verbal, physical or psychological abuse. Such emotionally heated events often take place in childhood. Sometimes just exposure to traumatic experience involving other people produces large negative effects. These old events remain imprinted in the nervous system. How can the child make sense or reconcile in her/his mind co-existence of care and respect with abuse and violence? What governs the spiritual world of humans? The child's world now is split on two parts. Most of the time people's behavior is governed by equality, care, respect, and peace in relation to each other.

However, this is only the external camouflage since the real structure or hierarchy of people is in the abilities of some to abuse and others to tolerate the abuses. This is where the real power or core of the relationship, in child's view, is hidden.

These social ideas provide a matrix (framework or cliché) that will be used later in order to relate, or judge, or evaluate other people and build new relationships with them using those old roles.

On a personal level, conscious thinking about old traumas can result in re- experience of anger, helplessness, guilt, resentment, alienation and hostility (as during the trauma). These toxic emotions can poison psychological well-being and breathing of the person years later.

We seek justice and revenge in relation to past abuses. No peace of mind seems possible unless the perpetrators repent and are duly punished. But the perpetrators can be far away and unconcerned with the past. We, on the other hand, carry the heavy burden of emotional hostility on our shoulders even when nobody is around. At other moments we abuse others without noticing it. Once the abuse started, it can spread like a domino effect: from generation to generation or like a growing and branching tree.

5.12 Do other factors also generate stress?

All other factors mentioned previously lead to chronic hyperventilation. Chronic hyperventilation causes the brain of modern man to be over-excited. As a result, people often perceive threats and become stressed, when there is no genuine reason. Stress, instead of being a healthy challenge, becomes another cause of chronic hyperventilation. In animals, stress also results in hyperventilation, together with other elements of the "fight-or-flight" response (e.g., hormonal rush). However, animals usually fight, or flee, seconds after the challenge. They exercise and their breathing gets back to normal sooner rather than later. Most modern humans, on the other hand, feel stressed and anxious, without getting involved in physical activity later.

Is it fair to claim that modern man experiences more stress now than our primitive predecessors did in the past? Many primitive people probably had daily situations when their lives were seriously threatened. Are there many people nowadays, who face death on a daily basis? Very few do. Hence, from an objective viewpoint, people in the past had much more stress. However, the excited mental states of modern people can make their lives too stressful and anxious due to over-reactions to ordinary and non-threatening situations.

This is an example of a vicious circle. Stress, along with other factors, causes chronic hyperventilation. In its turn, chronic hyperventilation impairs normal perception, resulting in more stress. This new stress can be generated even in non-violent situations.

5.13 Which factors are practically most important when we get sicker?

They are individual to the person and can vary over time for the same person. For example, a healthy young man, after graduation, may become less active physically. Breathing gets heavier. After some years he gradually gains weight.

That further intensifies breathing and lowers the CP. Later he starts breathing through his mouth and sleeping on his back. He becomes and feels more and more unwell. Presence of a childhood psycho trauma would be a great amplifier of these negative effects. Here, a combination of factors has gradually made his breathing heavier. If one wants to get back to the norm, to reverse the negative factors is the solution.

5.14 Do old movies and films show that breathing in the past was different?

You may notice the following differences.

1. People kept their mouths shut (except during speaking, eating, drinking, or when experiencing a strong surprise or awe).

2. People spent hours while reading, speaking, and working in the correct posture, which means a straight spine, shoulders back, and the chin up.

3. The gait and other body movements (like standing up, carrying objects, picking objects from the floor, bending, dancing, etc.) were done with a straight spine. Irrelevant muscles were relaxed. One can observe spontaneity, simplicity, effortlessness, co-ordination and grace in these actions.

4. There were no (or few) sighs, deep inhalations or exhalations, coughing, sneezing, etc.

5. The breathing of most people was invisible.

6. There were no deep inhalations before starting to speak or between phrases.

7. People's voices were deeper, more melodic, and rich in inner thoracic vibrations since normal breathing and higher CO2 values dilate air passages and relax vocal cords.

Be observant. Can you notice these differences in old movies and films?

Chapter 6. Buteyko trials and pilot studies

6.1 Work of Professor Buteyko and his colleagues

Professor Konstantin Buteyko (1923-2003) was a Soviet (Russian) medical doctor and clinical physician who devoted his life to the study of respiration.

When he was an Honors student of the First Moscow Medical Institute in the early 1950s, he observed that severely sick people usually had heavy breathing and that their breathing got even heavier when death approached. (You can visit any hospital to observe this simple fact.) The CP of terminally ill people gradually decreased: 5 s, 4, 3, 2, 1, and 0, when death occurred.

For several years in the 1960's, Dr. Buteyko was heading a project funded by the Ministry of Aviation and Space Research as a part of the program for launching first manned spaceships in the outer space. So, Dr. Buteyko was given a respiratory laboratory in Novosibirsk for this purpose. However, since he was also interested in diseases, he conducted many other studies. There he developed a system of breathing exercises and other auxiliary activities to restore normal breathing in his patients.

In 1985, the Soviet Health Ministry officially approved the Buteyko breathing method. It has been used by family doctors (or GPs) and breathing practitioners in Russia for more than 100,000 asthmatics, over 30,000 people with cardiovascular problems and many other patients. The Buteyko breathing method has saved the lives of thousands of people in the Soviet Union who were officially diagnosed as terminally ill.

The method has had several successful clinical trials (England, Australia, New Zealand, Ukraine, USSR). Practice shows that normalization of breathing for most people means to become disease-free. It is still unclear, due to our limited knowledge, which health problems can be treated and what the success rates for various health conditions are. In the meantime, let us consider these trials in more detail.

6.2 Clinical trials for asthmatics

In 2003 the Thorax Medical Journal published a report about the world's largest clinical trial, world-wide, of the Buteyko breathing method involving 600 adults with asthma (McGowan, 2003). It stated, "The participants involved in this study all experienced significant improvement in asthma with a reduction in symptoms, medication and improvement in quality of life". No improvements were found for the placebo and control groups.

It is probably not a great surprise for the reader that the quality of life became better for all those practicing the Buteyko method. As for medication, there are two common types of drugs used by asthmatics: reliever medication e.g., Ventolin and often preventer medication e.g., cortisol-based steroids. The use of reliever medication decreased about 50 times, preventer medication more than 12 times. The asthma symptoms' score decreased 50 times.

The trial was possible due to the heroic efforts of a clinical nurse and former University lecturer from Glasgow Jill McGowan, BIBH (Buteyko Institute of Breathing and Health). Before the beginning of the trial, she tried to get financial support from various organizations, funds and societies in the UK. After some unsuccessful attempts, she sold her house in order to raise money for the trial.

Later, she was awarded the Great Scot Award 2001 and the Pride of Britain Award 2002 for the outstanding results of the trial and her courage and devotion.

In the same year the New Zealand Medical Journal published an article about the result of another clinical trial for asthmatics conducted at the Gisborne Hospital (McHugh et al, 2003). The title of the article explains the results - Buteyko Breathing Technique for asthma: an effective intervention. Russell Stark, a Buteyko practitioner, taught the Buteyko group. The study was blinded, randomized and controlled. After 6 months, they reduced inhaled steroid use by 50% and ß2-agonist use by 85%. In the conclusion, the medical professionals wrote, "BBT [Buteyko breathing technique] is a safe and efficacious asthma management technique. BBT has clinical and potential pharmaco-economic benefits that merit further study".

In 2000, the Journal of Asthma reported: A clinical trial of the Buteyko Breathing Technique in asthma as taught by a Video (Opat et al, 2000).

Eighteen patients with mild to moderate asthma were taught the Buteyko method by a video and compared with 18 control subjects. The study found a significant improvement in the quality of life and a significant reduction in inhaled steroid use.

Two years earlier, the Medical Journal of Australia published a study Buteyko breathing techniques in asthma: a blinded randomised controlled trial (Bowler et al, 1998). This trial was conducted in Mater Hospital, Brisbane, Australia. There were 20 patients who had a long history of asthma and significant medication. In 3 months, they decreased the use of bronchodilators by 90%, inhaled steroids by 50%. The symptoms' score was improved by 71%.

Currently, 6 most successful controlled randomized clinical trials on asthma were conducted using the Buteyko breathing technique. The organizers and participants of these trials were located in Australia, New Zealand and the UK.

6.3 Russian and Ukrainian trials on patients with liver problems, AIDS, radiation disease, childhood asthma, adult asthma and heart disease

The Soviet health care system, for political and social reasons, had always been more centralized than Western ones. Innovations in medicine were usually introduced by the Soviet authorities and health care bureaucracy. New ideas and drugs were often tested in hospitals and research Institutes, which provided higher authorities with reports about the results. In the West, as we know, results of scientific studies or trials are usually published in journals. While the Soviet approach was different, the reliability of their information was comparable.

Directors, managers and project leaders of corresponding organizations and departments put their signatures to official reports about such Soviet trials and their approbations. These people were personally responsible for the trustworthiness of the results and their names and copies of the relevant documents, related to the Buteyko trials as well, are still archived in Russia and Ukraine.

In 1991, the Scientific Research Institute of Epidemiology and Infectious Diseases, named after L. V. Gromashevsky in Kiev, Ukraine conducted two clinical trials using the Buteyko method. One trial was for 30 patients diagnosed with acute and chronic hepatitis and cirrhosis of the liver. Twenty-eight patients had remissions of their symptoms while twenty-five showed improvements in their blood test results.

The second trial involved 7 patients with AIDS. Progression of this disease is usually accompanied by a variety of symptoms and complaints in the digestive, immune, cardiovascular, respiratory, hormonal and other systems. The official documents of the Institute provided information about the patients' quality of life such as emotional stability, irritability, panic attacks, chronic fatigue, insomnia, digestive complaints and some other factors. All symptoms were relieved with no side effects due to breathing retraining.

One year earlier, another Ukrainian trial in Kiev tested the effects of the Buteyko method on 50 patients with radiation sickness as a result of Chernobyl's nuclear plant disaster. The work took place in Shevchenko's Central Hospital. Eighty-two percent of the patients showed considerable improvement in blood analysis, cardiovascular parameters (blood pressure, pulse, etc.), efficiency of the digestive system, and reduction in medication. No cases of side effects or complications due to the breathing exercises were reported.

Breathing Slower and Less: The Greatest Health Discovery Ever

In 1981, the Sechenov's Medical Institute in Moscow conducted a trial for 52 severely sick children, aged 3-15, with regular asthma attacks (once per day or more). All had problems breathing through their noses, suffered from heart palpitations, and used bronchodilators. In 1-5 days, the patients were able to stop the attacks of asthma and cough, to unblock their noses and to prevent wheezing, using the method. Observations over 1-3 months showed considerable improvements (cessation of heavy attacks or a total disappearance of the symptoms) in 83%, and some improvement (fewer heavy attacks and considerable reduction in medication) in the remaining 17%. Their average CP increased from 4 to 30 s.

The very first pilot trial took place in 1968 in the Institute of Pulmonology, Leningrad, USSR. Fifty patients had severe bronchial asthma, hypertension and angina pectoris. All of them had many years of heavy medication. Most had hormonal deficiencies and organic complications. Forty nine (out of 50) patients discarded their medication or significantly decreased its use.

Apart from these trials, Soviet medical professionals who practiced the Buteyko method had conferences where they shared their experiences. Two such meetings in Moscow and Krasnoyarsk in 1988 resulted in 30 published reports. The reported number of treated people, according to the conference proceedings, totaled over 3,000. Although most of them had respiratory (asthma, bronchitis, rhinitis, etc.) and cardiovascular (hypertension, angina pectoris, ischemia, etc.) problems, hundreds were treated and got relief from arthritis, osteoporosis, epilepsy, ulcers, gastritis, kidney stone problems, hepatitis, endometriosis, skin diseases (e.g., dermatitis, psoriasis, eczema), and some other conditions.

Typically, over 90% of the patients reported that their symptoms were either somewhat improved or considerably improved. Virtually all the medical professionals acknowledged in their articles that those patients who reduced their breathing and, hence, achieved large CPs significantly improved their state of health.

None of all these trials or reports revealed any complications or side effects due to the Buteyko breathing method. (Indeed, how could the fundamental physiological norms harm the human organism?) This testifies to the professionalism of the Buteyko doctors and teachers, since there are many important practical rules.

6.4 Best cancer-cure clinical trial ever used the Buteyko method

Dr. Buteyko's pupil, Dr. Sergey Paschenko organized the most successful clinical trial in history of cancer research. The trial was conducted on 120 people with metastatic breast cancer. When a clinical trial on cancer manages to reduce mortality by 20-25%, it is considered as a major breakthrough in cancer research. In fact, only some (not all) studies that tested effects of chemotherapy and radiation on patients with metastatic cancer could achieve such success (20-25% less mortality in 3 or 5 years).

However, in this phenomenal clinical trial, the group that practiced breathing exercises had nearly **6 times less mortality** during the following 3 years. You could not find anything similar in the whole history of cancer research. Most successful trials that proved efficiency of surgery and chemotherapy had only about10-20% reduction in mortality. More details about this trial are in my book "Doctors Who Cure Cancer".

6.5 Were there any clinical trials or studies for heart patients?

There were no special trials for heart patients. During the very first pilot trial of the Buteyko method in 1968 in Leningrad, many patients (out of 50) had severe forms of the heart disease and the results of the breathing retraining therapy were remarkable.

Later, clinical research by Professor Buteyko and his colleagues resulted in several publications about heart disease. For example, they found a linear relationship between blood levels of cholesterol and the CP in those who tend to develop cholesterol deposits. The higher the CP, the lower the blood cholesterol.

Normalization of breathing, as their practice showed, caused elimination of symptoms and normalization of blood levels of cholesterol and normal blood pressure. More research and more clinical trials and studies are needed in order to substantiate this effect and identify the mechanisms of these processes.

References for Chapter 6

Bowler SD, Green A, Mitchell CA, Buteyko breathing techniques in asthma: a blinded randomized controlled trial, Med J of Australia 1998; 169: 575-578.

Cooper S, Oborne J, Newton S, Harrison V, Thompson Coon J, Lewis S, Tattersfield A, Effect of two breathing exercises (Buteyko and pranayama) in asthma: a randomized controlled trial, Thorax 2003; 58: 674-679.

Cowie RL, Conley DP, Underwood MF, Reader PG, A randomized controlled trial of the Buteyko technique as an adjunct to conventional management of asthma, Respir Med. 2008 May; 102(5): 726-732.

Douglas CG, Haldane JS, The regulation of normal breathing, Journal of Physiology 1909; 38: p. 420-440.

Hasselbalch, Biochem Zeitschr, 1912, XLVI, p. 416.

McGowan J, Health education in asthma management - Does the Buteyko Institute Method make a difference? Thorax December 2003, Vol. 58, sup. III, p.28.

McHugh P, Aitcheson, Duncan B, Houghton F, Buteyko Breathing Technique for asthma: an effective intervention, New Zealand Medical Journal 12 December 2003, 116 (1187): p. 710-716.

Opat AJ, Cohen MM, Bailey MJ, Abramson MJ, A clinical trial of the Buteyko Breathing Technique in asthma as taught by a Video, Journal of Asthma 2000; 37(7): p. 557-564.

Slader CA, Reddel HK, Spencer LM, Belousova EG, Thien FC, ArmourCL, Bosnic-Anticevich SZ, Jenkins CR, Impact of breathing exercises on asthma symptoms and control, Thorax Journal 2006, 000: 1-7.

Chapter 7. Questions and answers about the Buteyko method and breathing retraining

7.1 Does the efficiency of oxygen extraction depend on breathing?

Chronic hyperventilators (e.g., with CPs from 15 to 25 s) use only about 10-20% of inhaled oxygen at rest, the remaining 80-90% O2 is exhaled! People considered normal by medical standards retain only about a quarter (25%) of the oxygen that they inhale. Their lungs are more efficient at extracting oxygen.

Those healthy people, who breathe little (4 l/min or less), can extract up to 30- 35% of the oxygen they inhale. In addition, they inhale much fewer toxic fumes, dust particles, pollens, and other dangerous substances. This is another reason to breathe less.

Finally, as it was quoted above, several Western studies found that blood flow and oxygenation of many vital organs are proportional to body CO2 concentrations. Tissue hypoxia of vital organs is a normal feature of chronic hyperventilation.

7.2 I have been taught that yogi and very healthy people have deep breathing and that deep breathing is good for the health. Is that wrong?

Very healthy people (over 2 min CP) have a very slow breathing pattern at rest. They are breathing only about 3-4 times per minute at rest inhaling almost up to 700-900 milliliters of air per one breath (for example, during sleep). People with about 60 s CP often breathe about 500-600 milliliters per breath with a breathing frequency about 6-9 times per minute. Sick people usually breathe deeper; that is, they breathe up to 1 liter per breath and do that 15-25 times per minute or even more.

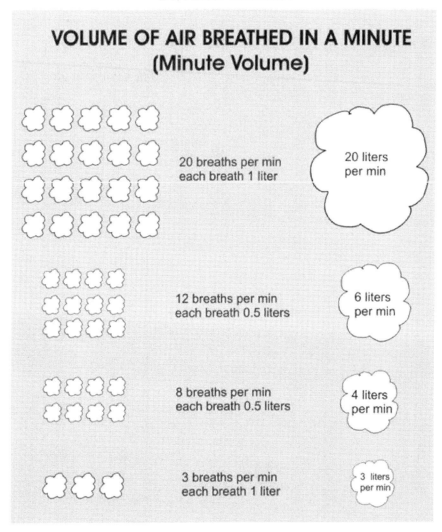

VOLUME OF AIR BREATHED IN A MINUTE (Minute Volume)

20 breaths per min
each breath 1 liter

20 liters per min

12 breaths per min
each breath 0.5 liters

6 liters per min

8 breaths per min
each breath 0.5 liters

4 liters per min

3 breaths per min
each breath 1 liter

3 liters per min

Hence, both very healthy and sick people usually have deep breathing in comparison with standards of normal breathing or official medical/physiological standards. However, very healthy people have higher than normal CO_2 concentrations while sick people have lower than normal CO_2 levels.

Many teachers and practitioners of Western yoga schools have been promoting the idea of the importance of deep breathing. Moreover, their practices often encourage deep and fast breathing. In terms of

CO_2, such breathing can cause, and does cause degenerative physiological changes. Facts show (see the picture) that in order to become healthy, most people need, firstly, to learn shallow breathing. Indeed, their breathing is too deep, but normal breathing is shallower.

Only later, one may try to develop very slow yogic breathing in order to approach ideal health.

7.3 Can I try voluntary hyperventilation in order to feel its effects?

Russian Buteyko doctors have used voluntary hyperventilation for more than 30 years in order to show patients the destructive effects of deep breathing and its symptoms. If you are in good health, you can try many (up to 100) deep and fast successive breaths. "Let us have deep breathing for the last time," as some Russian breathing teachers say. People with low CPs often get exhausted after 30 or 50 fast and deep breaths. Asthmatics and people with heart disease experience symptoms of those diseases well before their hundredth inhalation.

Warning. It is better to do this test under supervision. This test can be dangerous for people with severe forms of diseases. Generally, the sicker the person, the more dangerous the test is. Stop at the first signs of strange or unusual symptoms.

Remember these symptoms. Now you can prevent development of acute episodes or attacks by using reduced breathing. If that is not possible through reduced breathing, then you may need half dose of your medication.

7.4 I like to go to yoga classes and swimming. Are they good for my breathing and health?

Buteyko practitioners measure the effects of various activities by testing eventual changes in automatic breathing. What are the long-term effects? Practically, you can do that by measuring your CP before and after the activity. First, rest for 5-7 min just before your yoga class or swimming. Then determine your CP before you begin the activity. Later, repeat the test after you have rested from doing the activity. If your new CP gets higher, this activity is useful for your health. If not, then we do not recommend it to our students. The same relates to yoga classes, swimming and other activities.

Note that if your activity is physically demanding (like 1 hour of swimming or running), you may need 0.5 - 1 hour of rest before the second CP measurement. This break is necessary for stabilization of your metabolism. Immediately after rigorous activities, the CP is often low, but hours later it gets larger.

7.5 Are there many activities and health therapies that improve breathing?

Yes. Physical activity with a closed mouth is very beneficial for most people.

That relates to people whose CPs are above 20 s and who feel fit to exercise.

When one's CP is below 20 s, walking is an excellent exercise. "*Walking is man's best medicine*", as suggested by Greek physician Hippocrates (460 BC - 377 BC).

Practicing relaxation, meditation, prayer, yoga postures, tai chi, Alexander technique, acupuncture, osteopathy, herbal science, colonic irrigation, elimination of nutritional problems and deficiencies and many other therapies and methods can double or improve the CP in some people by 5-10 s. Just measure it. However, the efficiency of these methods is variable and often depends on current CP and other health factors of the person.

7.6 Flyers and websites of Buteyko practitioners rarely say anything about the breathing exercises. Are there secrets?

No. There are no secrets. The basic idea behind the breathing exercises is to practice shallow (or reduced) breathing with slight air hunger while having correct posture and while relaxing all of the muscles, including the diaphragm, during exhalation. However, it usually takes about 7-10 hours (or 5-7 lessons) for a practitioner to explain the basics of the method and details of the breathing exercises, observe how they are done, correct mistakes of the student, and provide further guidance and support.

In the 1960's Dr. Buteyko wanted to provide Soviet patients with instructions about his breathing method. He wrote a manual that explained in detail practical steps for doing the breathing exercises. The manual was distributed among many patients. However, Dr. Buteyko and his colleagues found, to their surprise, that less than 1% of patients were able to learn the method from the manual. It was a disaster. Meanwhile, his breathing instructors were able to achieve over 90% success rate by teaching the method directly to their students/patients.

Are there some special personality traits that help me with learning the method? The main requirement is personal determination and self-discipline. Technically, much depends on a person's ability to feel own breathing. Sit down and try to listen to your breathing for a minute. Are you able to feel the movement of air in your nose? In your throat? In your bronchi? Do you feel how your lungs are filled with air? Do you feel the movements of your diaphragm? It will be easier and faster for you to learn the method, if you answer "yes" to most of these questions. However, even when people can't feel their breathing, they are still able to learn and master the method.

7.7 Can I get healthier by practicing breath holding or delays in breathing?

A few people can achieve some success, but this route can be risky. For many people, delays in breathing, without an understanding of the method, would result in more muscular tension and stress with deeper breathing later. Moreover, if you have certain health problems, then some types of breath-holds can worsen your health.

For example, for some people, long delays or breath holds and strong air hunger can lead to unpleasant or even dangerous side effects, such as headaches, quick hormonal changes, changes in blood pressure, or intensified digestion with burping and "flare-ups". Practitioners know these concerns.

7.8 Is it useful to practice slow breathing since healthy people have small breathing frequency?

Some modern hatha yoga teachers use slow breathing practices (e.g., pranayama). However, the Buteyko breathing method does not use counting of breathing frequency. The method is based on having restricted inhalation, relaxed passive exhalation and light air hunger disregarding the number of breaths per minute.

7.9 How soon can I achieve normal breathing and a 60 s CP?

Practice shows that this process is slow and usually takes, with the application of the optimal breathing program, weeks or months for young people, and months or years for adults. There are also many other factors involved, including your determination, devotion, initial health status, available time, and other conditions (like job, exercise, and diet).

7.10 Do many people achieve a 60 s CP? How far do most people progress?

Not many. People use the Buteyko breathing method for various purposes. A few people are satisfied with basic breathing control. Simple breathing exercises help them to prevent acute episodes, like asthma or heart attacks, or, for example, to unblock the nose. These people practice breathing exercises mainly during these emergency episodes. The method is used instead of taking medication. Such students often have low CPs (about 20-25 s or less). This is Level 1 training.

Most people go further and experience improvements in their quality of life as described above. They can reach, for example, 30-40 s daily CPs after some months (with 20+ for typical morning CPs), as was done by many during clinical trials. Such CPs correspond to Level 2 and permit them to have a better quality of life usually with no medication.

Why do they not progress further, to Level 3 (over 60 s CP)? Firstly, when people achieve significant improvements, they get busy with their lives and practice less. Secondly, it is usually not easy to go beyond a 40 s CP. One needs commitment, perseverance, self-discipline and patience for many months or years. Thirdly, many Buteyko teachers do not encourage and explain to their students that it is possible to progress further. Finally, very few teachers know methods and techniques that are required to get 60+ s CP 24/7.

7.11 Are there many people who claim that breathing retraining was useless for them?

I still have to hear or meet a person who increased his or her CP 2-3 times or get it up to 60 s CP without experiencing any changes. (Probably, this is impossible physiologically.) However, sometimes individuals try to manipulate their breathing, do some exercises, but, unfortunately, cannot achieve any positive long-term changes in their breathing due to various obstacles and mistakes.

7.12 How do I know that a certain breathing teacher is good for me?

Professor Buteyko established the requirement for Soviet doctors to have at least 60 s CP. Buteyko thought that only those doctors who normalized their own breathing should teach the method. This is a wise criterion. Russian doctors are still trying to keep this standard.

Western breathing teachers often have less than 60 s CPs (e.g., 30 s). Is it a big problem? No, if you want to achieve the same level, as your possible breathing teacher. He or she can guide you till his or her own CP. Western breathing teachers do great job in saving lives and health restoration.

If you intend to have vibrant health (over 60 s CP), then the CP of your teacher can be the factor. Practice shows that usually breathing teachers train their students till the same CP level as they have. Larger CPs demand clearer and more detailed understanding of the Buteyko method.

7.13 Why did Professor Buteyko introduce his norms for breathing?

Let us look at the history of official Western breathing standards. The current norms at rest for a 70-kg man can be found in medical and physiological textbooks: CO_2 - 40 mm Hg (or about 5.3% at sea level), ventilation - 6 l/min, the CP - 40 s.

How did the main parameter "40 mm Hg CO_2" appear? Through experimentation, it was established by the famous British researchers Charles G.

Douglas and John S. Haldane from Oxford University about a century ago. Their results were published in the article The regulation of normal breathing by the Journal of Physiology (Douglas & Haldane, 1909). The investigators analyzed arterial blood gases of staff members at Oxford University, including scientists and support personnel, and found an average. It is possible to argue that even during those times many University workers had a sedentary life style with little physical activity. Hence, their usual CO_2 concentrations could be lower than those for most healthy people. Indeed, another old study by the also famous Karl Albert Hasselbalch had about 45 mm Hg as an average value for breathing at rest (Hasselbalch, 1912).

Some textbooks define hyperventilation as a state with less than 40 mm Hg CO_2 while others (and most) less than 35 mm Hg. More recent textbooks often have 8-9 l/min as "normal values". Some modern clinical studies used the CO_2 values of volunteers as a standard for comparison with sick people and found small differences between groups. In some recent studies, CO_2 values of "healthy volunteers" can be as low as 34-36 mm Hg. If most modern people are chronic hyperventilators (according to official standards), should new average values become our new standards?

From a practical viewpoint, Russian medical research indicates that people with 30-40 s CP still can have certain serious health problems, many of which disappear with further progress in breathing parameters. Sixty seconds CPs and 6.5% CO_2 (or about 46% mm Hg CO_2), on the other hand, are indicators of vibrant health in which many modern diseases are impossible. If disease-free health is the goal of modern medicine, would it not make sense to accept Buteyko's standards that provide a guarantee of excellent health?

7.14 Is it possible that some people can have large CPs while still having health problems or being sick?

Situations with unusually large CPs are very rare, but they were described in medical literature. Some brain surgeries involve the medulla of the brain (the location of the breathing center) or the nerve cells that control respiratory muscles. In these cases, CO_2 sensitivity can decrease or totally disappear causing artificially large CPs.

In real life, people with, for example, sleep apnea and emphysema usually have CPs that are slightly higher than the CPs that one could expect visually estimating their breathing patterns.

Some people are genetically predisposed to cardiovascular problems. If such people frequently perform very long breath holds, it is possible that their small blood vessels have not been able to adjust (or dilate) due to this sudden transition to higher CO_2 levels and that may result in some abnormalities in, for example, blood perfusion. This results in abnormally high CPs.

7.15 What are the changes in breathing during breathing retraining?

CO2 is the main regulator of breathing. It tells how much one breathes. Here is a simplified picture based on CO2 effects. We know that sick people chronically breathe too heavily. Their breathing center is preset to a low CO2 value. In order to retrain their breathing, they need to gradually reset their breathing center to higher CO2 levels. Thus, day after day, week after week and month after month, they gradually readjust their breathing center to breathing less and less air. Their CP gets higher and higher. Some days it may drop. However, week after week there is a general progress, e.g., by 2-4 s or more. For some people, especially obese, the CP increases only by about 1 s in a week. Whatever the rate of the progress, persistence and self-discipline pay back with easier breathing.

7.16 How much time should I practice daily in order to progress with breathing?

Usually 1 hour of breathing exercises per day is enough. This time is divided among 2-4 or several breathing sessions, about 10-30 min long, depending on your individual plan and breathing exercises as suggested by your practitioner. If one devotes more time (e.g., 3-5 hours per day), the progress is faster and the results are often spectacular.

Apart from the breathing sessions, you need to be conscious to other common sense factors, like keeping your mouth closed, not overeating, not sleeping on the back, etc. Altogether, you need, at least "one hour plus". That means 1 hour of your time for breathing sessions with some additional common-sense steps and activities of the program. People do not regret the time spent. Reduced requirements for sleep and other improvements in quality of life quickly make up for all initial investments of time and energy.

The Buteyko method is still changing and evolving so that people can improve their health with minimum efforts and get busy with their lives. To achieve this goal, breathing teachers share their ideas with each other.

7.17 Are there any age requirements?

As soon as people can understand and follow simple instructions, they can learn the method. According to Russian practice, that relates even to patients with the initial stages of schizophrenia. Children from 3 years old and above can also understand the method and its instructions. However, as a requirement, parents or caretakers of these children should also practice the method for better results.

There are special methods for younger children (0-2 years) as well.

7.18 If I have achieved normal breathing and a 60 s CP, should I practice these breathing exercises for the rest of my life?

Above I have tried to show that high CPs were human norms centuries ago.

Those people did not practice any special breathing exercises. Why did they have good breath holding abilities then? Many conditions were different, but physical exercise was probably the most important factor. Most people in the past were physically active for many hours per day. Similarly, if you have normal breathing and 4-5 hours of physical activity every day, you will be generously rewarded with excellent health and well-being. And that is not hard for them, since people with large CPs enjoy physical activity.

Russian practical experience shows that having 4-5 hours of daily exercise is usually enough to preserve normal breathing and a normal CP. If people cannot exercise and want to have normal breathing, then, as Russians believe, they need to continue to practice the breathing exercises on a daily basis.

7.19 Do all people need this large amount of physical activity?

Sick people need physical activity to stimulate the lymphatic system. There are many other physiological reasons why we need physical activity. Shaking of the body (as during jumping or riding in train) intensifies biochemical processes. The hormonal profile can normalize. Some useful chemicals can be produced.

However, physical exercise is also useful to counteract the muscular tension due to past psychological traumas, if the person cannot let them go.

Some people hold the past negative emotions within. They are seeking revenge and want to get even. They are still not at peace with the past remembering and bringing to others anger, helplessness, guilt, resentment, alienation and hostility.

Their new relationships suffer due to unresolved past traumas. Such people need more physical activity and/or breathing exercises in order to eliminate muscular tension and accumulation of negative energy. Physical activity helps to discharge the negative energy.

If a person can let those traumas and negative emotions go, then he/she can go on with the life while having clear minds, cheerful mood and easy breathing.

Practice shows that vibrant health is possible with little physical activity.

7.20 How can I let them go?

Note that I am not talking about forgetting about those events. I also do not mean condoning or excusing the perpetrators. In fact, in some cases, it could be better for all involved sides to take legal actions against the perpetrators.

There is no a single side that is winning from having these negative emotions (anger, helplessness, guilt, resentment, alienation and hostility). They generate further alienation, self-destruction and hostility. Even our new relationships suffer. Many people carry this heavy burden of the past forever. Our culture particularly encourages such macho-behavior in males.

There are various methods and techniques that were developed by humanity in order to deal with this huge and old problem present, to a certain degree, in every human being. Virtually all sources in this area are labeled under the title "forgiveness" (or letting it go). If you are determined to forgive somebody, find books or articles. Some useful information can be found here: www.forgivenessweb.com. You can also download for free a good book *"Why forgive?"* from www.bruderhof.com.

More radical and fast solution of past traumas is the New Decision Therapy developed by Kandis Blakely (USA). There are now many NDT practitioners in various countries who help to forgive others and selves. An average session only requires 60-70 minutes instead of years of psychoanalysis or other techniques.

7.21 Does the Buteyko method help with all diseases?

The Buteyko breathing method will help to improve health for anybody with symptoms of chronic hyperventilation and small CPs (e.g., 30 s or less). As for some specific diseases and health conditions, more research is needed to have a clear picture about the breathing retraining effects. It is not necessary to feel or to be sick in order to learn the Buteyko method. There are many people in Russia who have learned the method for spiritual reasons.

7.22 Is CO2 the only reason for the success of the Buteyko method?

CO2 is the most known and investigated factor that relates to breathing and the Buteyko method. There are many other factors that are known to students and practitioners.

The Buteyko method also includes, for example, psychological factors. The students learn how to stop their symptoms and prevent attacks, how to react to stress and other factors that cause hyperventilation. Hence, the students acquire a sense of control over their health. Helplessness and depression are no longer the parameters that define the course of their diseases.

Nasal breathing helps the body to use its own nitric oxide that is produced in nasal passages. The roles and some important effects of this hormone have been discovered very recently and there are still many questions in relation to this substance.

Emphasis on diaphragmatic breathing and relaxation of chest breathing muscles should favor elimination of possible abnormalities in regulation of breathing by the autonomic nervous system. Activity of the chest breathing muscles at rest often points to sympathetic dominance since chest muscles get active during both exercise and hyperventilation. While the Buteyko method is not focused on slow diaphragmatic breathing pattern, this pattern gradually appears by itself, for example, during sleep. Diaphragmatic breathing promotes natural lymphatic drainage of the nodes located under the diaphragm.

Passive relaxed exhalation during the breathing sessions should also have good effects on the balance between parasympathetic and sympathetic nervous systems. These systems are often out of balance for many diseases, like asthma, heart disease, chronic fatigue, cancer and many other health problems.

Deliberate attention to posture and relaxation of body muscles should also influence the autonomous nervous system. When we relax and breathing is lighter, we again pacify the overexcited sympathetic nervous system. It is often chronically over-active due to the fight-or-flight mode induced by hyperventilation. Healing and tissue repair, on the other hand, are more active when the parasympathetic system is dominant.

Reduced breathing decreases levels of free (unbound) oxygen in the lungs and blood creating temporary hypoxia. This mild hypoxia, first, appears in the lungs and, later, in blood. However, the CP increases in minutes due to the Bohr effect, vasodilation and other processes. Hence, tissue oxygenation is improved, but less oxygen is in the free state. Free oxygen in our bodies generates free radicals causing cellular damage and aging, especially for lungs. This damage is stronger during hyperventilation.

It is difficult to tell at the present time what the isolated effects of these factors are. Clearly, they are individual. Can the various effects of the Buteyko method be separated? Probably yes, for example, using CO_2 injections or CO_2 chambers or submarines with special air.

More practical work, tests, and biochemical research is required to investigate the effects of breathing retraining on people with various health problems and conditions.

7.23 What are the typical long-term results (after year or two)?

After more than 10 years of clinical experience, I realized that it is very common for many students to get their best results in 2-3 months of practice, but later, since they feel much better, do not experience symptoms, and stop taking medication, most students reduce amounts of their breathing exercises without increasing physical activity. This causes a drop in their CPs after several months of practice and during following years.

Here is a graph that reflects these changes in the **morning CP**.

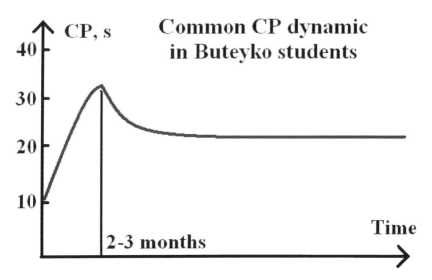

Therefore, most students still have better health. They usually do not require any medication, but I cannot say that they enjoy really good health.

7.25 What are the main methods to maintain high CPs?

The Buteyko breathing exercises were created for sick and severely sick people most of whom were hospitalized. According to Dr. Buteyko, the main method that helps to maintain great health and high CP is physical exercise.

Based on my experience with hundreds of breathing students, here is the link that reflects effects of exercise on one's morning CP.

Duration of physical exercise per day	Maximum body O2 expected
0 min	15 s
30 min	20 s
60 min	25 s
1 hour of devoted PE + 1 hour others	30 s
1.5 hour of devoted PE + 1 hour others	35 s
2 hours of devoted PE + 1 hour others	Up to 2-3 min

Table note. "PE" means physical exercise. "1.5 hour of devoted PE + 1 hour others" means that the person spends 1.5 hour on devoted physical exercise (for example, 2 daily jogging sessions of 45 min each) and also gets 1 hour of walking throughout the day.

Many sick people, especially city dwellers, often have less than 20 min of physical exercise per day. (These 20 minutes include walking within the house, to the car, while shopping, etc.). Their body and brain oxygenation is, at best, according to this table, about 18 seconds due to habitual chest breathing, mouth breathing and overbreathing (breathing more than the medical norm at rest).

If a person with over 20 second CP devotes 1 hour to rigorous physical activity with nose breathing only, they can finally get stabilized, over a period of some days, at the level of about 25 seconds of body O2. Usually such people naturally get about 30 min of light exercise throughout the day (e.g., walking here and there).

Having more than 2 hours of daily physical activity is generally sufficient to get or maintain any body-oxygen levels.

Elderly people often require less physical exercise than suggested by the Table above. For example, a 60+ or 70+ years old person may require only 1 hour of devoted exercise and 1 hour of walking to get any body oxygenation, provided that there are few, if any, negative effects due to other lifestyle risk factors.

Teenagers and young people in their 20s and 30s sometimes may require more physical activity to achieve main benefits of physical exercise and the corresponding body O2 numbers shown in the Table.

Note that it is assumed here that other factors, including breath-work, sleep hygiene, diet, nutritional deficiencies, thermoregulation, daily work, and posture, do not produce negative effects on morning oxygenation.

Note about recovery from chronic diseases. People with pathological tissue changes (inflammation, tumors, deposits, lymphomas, granulomas, and so on) generally cannot get even 25 s oxygenation without additional physical exercise.

7.26 Are there many benefits of having high morning CPs?

In a long run, most Western people, as it was mentioned above, get about 20-25 s for their morning CPs. These are good results due to reduction in symptoms and greatly improved life quality. However, main benefits due to breathing retraining take place at higher CP numbers.

Here is a short summary of some natural changes that are very common due to breathing retraining and getting over 50 s for the morning CP.

Lifestyle factor:	Body oxygen < 30 s	Body oxygen > 50 s
Energy level	Medium, low, or very low	High
Desire to exercise	Not strong, but possible	Craving and joy of exercise
Intensive exercise with nose breathing	Hard or impossible	Easy and effortless
Typical mind states	Confusion, anxiety, depression	Focus, concentration, clarity
Craving for coffee, sugar and junk foods	Present	Absent
Addictions to smoking, alcohol, and drugs	Possible	Absent
Desire to eat raw foods	Weak and rare	Very common and natural
Correct posture	Rare and requires efforts	Natural and automatic
Sleep	Often of poor quality; > 7 hours	Excellent quality; < 5 hours naturally

Appendix 1. How to find the CP using other breath holding time tests

Handbook of physiology (Mithoefer, 1965), after analyzing numerous relevant publications, suggested the following proportions for BHT (breath holding time) measurements (Mithoefer, 1965). If BHT after full inhalation is 100%; then BHT after normal inhalation is 55%; BHT after normal exhalation (the CP) is 40%; BHT after full exhalation is 24%. Taking an additional full exhalation or inhalation before starting the test increases BHT by about 5 or 15% respectively for each full maneuver. This information allows us to compare different BHT tests done during almost a century of clinical investigations. In order to do that, any other test will be changed to our standard, the CP (control pause).

Mithoefer JC, Breath holding. In: Handbook of physiology, Respiration, Washington, DC: American Physiological Society, 1965, sect. 3, vol. 2, chapter 38: 1011-1026.

BHT after full inhalation vs. CP

Based on these results, we can calculate that BHT after full inhalation is 2.5 times larger than the CP. Therefore, if you try to measure your stress-free breath holding time after full inhalation, you need to divide this result by 2.5 in order to get your real CP. For example, if yourBHT after full inhalation is 50 seconds, your CP is 20 seconds.

BHT after normal inhalation vs. CP

BHT after normal inhalation is nearly 1.4 times greater than the CP. For example, if your BHT after normal inhalation is 33 seconds, your CP is 24 seconds.

BHT after full exhalation vs. CP

If you do the maximum outhale (trying to empty the lungs) before the stress-free breath holding time test, then your result will be 10/6 times less than your CP. For example, with 12 seconds for BHT after full exhalation, your CP is about 20 seconds.

Note that people have different lung volumes and various breathing patterns. As a result, all these calculations are approximate. However, experience shows that among all these results for the BHT test, the CP is the most accurate measurement that reflects body oxygenation and overall health.

Appendix 2. Summary and explanation of normal respiratory and some related values

Normal parameters of different lung volumes

IC - Inspiratory capacity (difference between maximum lung volume and normal expiration) 3600 ml

ERV - Expiratory reserve volume (air volume which can be exhaled after normal expiration) 1200 ml

VC - Vital capacity (difference between maximum inhalation and maximum exhalation) 4800 ml

RV - Residual volume (air volume left in the lungs at full exhalation) 1200 ml

FRC - Functional residual capacity (volume of air in the lungs at normal expiration) 2400 ml

TLC - Total lung capacity (maximum air volume in the lungs at full inhalation) 6000 ml

Normal parameters of lung ventilation

Vt - Tidal volume (air volume breathed in during a single breath): 500 ml

Rf - Respiratory frequency (number of breathing cycles per minute): 12 breaths/min

MV - Minute volume (air volume breathed in and out during one minute): 6,000 ml/min

VA - Alveolar ventilation (air volume breathed in and out of the alveolar space in one minute): 4200 ml/min

Vd - Dead space volume (air volume in airways that does not exchange its oxygen with blood): 150-200 ml

MVV - Maximum voluntary ventilation (the largest air volume that can be moved into and out of the lungs in 1 minute by voluntary efforts): 170 L/min

FEV - Forced expiratory volume (air volume that can be forcefully expired in 1 or 3 sec divided by the vital capacity): 83% or 97%, respectively

Work of quiet breathing (amount of energy spent on quiet breathing at rest): 0.5 kg*m/min

Maximum work of breathing (maximum amount of energy that can be spent on breathing): 10 kg*m/min

Maximum inspiratory and expiratory pressures (maximum pressure gradients that can be voluntary created between the lungs and the outer air): 60-100 mm Hg

% saturation of hemoglobin with oxygen and amount of dissolved oxygen at different O2 pressures

For blood with 15 g/dl of hemoglobin, 38 degrees temperature, and 7.40 pH:

PO$_2$ mm Hg	% saturation of Hb	Dissolved O$_2$, ml/dl
30	57 %	0.09
40	75 %	0.12
50	84 %	0.15
60	90 %	0.18
70	93 %	0.21
80	95 %	0.24
90	97 %	0.27
100	98 %	0.30

support@

Normal gas content of the arterial blood

With 95 mm Hg O2 pressure, 40 mm Hg CO2 pressure, 15 g/dl of hemoglobin:

O2: 0.29 ml/dl dissolved; 19.5 ml/dl combined

CO2: 2.62 ml/dl dissolved; 46.4 ml/dl combined

N2: 0.98 ml/dl dissolved; 0 ml/dl combined.

Normal gas content of the venous blood

With 40 mm Hg O2 pressure, 46 mm Hg CO2 pressure, 15 g/dl of hemoglobin):

O2: 0.12 ml/dl dissolved; 15.1 ml/dl combined

CO2: 2.98 ml/dl dissolved; 49.7 ml/dl combined

N2: 0.98 ml/dl dissolved; 0 combined.

Normal components of worsupport@k of quiet breathing

Non-elastic work: 35%, including viscous resistance (7%) and airway resistance (28%) Elastic work: 65%.

Normal gas exchange parameters at sea level

Composition of outer air O_2 - Oxygen 158 mm Hg (20.9%) CO_2 - Carbon dioxide 0.3 mm Hg (0.04%) H_2O - Water 5.7 mm Hg (0.75%) N_2 - Nitrogen 596 mm Hg (78.4%)support@

Composition of the expired air O_2 - Oxygen 116 mm Hg (15.3%) CO_2 - Carbon dioxide 32 mm Hg (4.2%) H_2O - Water 47 mm Hg (6.2%) N_2 - Nitrogen 565 mm Hg (74.3%)

Composition of the alveolar air O_2 - support@Oxygen 100 mm Hg (13.2%) CO_2 - Carbon dioxide 40 mm Hg (5.3%) H_2O - Water 47 mm Hg (6.2%) N_2 - Nitrogen 573 mm Hg (75.4%)

Composition of the arterial blood O_2 - Oxygen 95 mm Hg (11.6%) CO_2 - Carbon dioxide 40 mm Hg (5.3%)

Composition of the venous blood O_2 - Oxygen 40 mm Hg (5.3%) CO_2 - Carbon dioxide 46 mm Hg (6

More details related to parameters of normal breathing can be found in the big book "Normal Breathing; The Key To Vital Health".

* These values are typically quoted as normal for a 70-kg man in medical and physiological textbooks.

Appendix 3. Clinical effects of the Buteyko method (or breathing retraining) on common health problems

These are typical results that are expected with most people, often over 90% of all breathing students.

Respiratory conditions

● Asthma
- An immediate decrease and, later, complete elimination of medication.
- Increase in the CP is accompanied by normalization of immunity.
- With the increased CP, allergic reactions become less severe and the number of allergens, which can provoke asthma attacks, decreases.
- Improved physical endurance and improved quality of life.
- Avoidance of triggers and high CPs (over 35 s 24/7) for 2-3 weeks lead to complete disappearance of allergies, disappearance of swelling and inflammation in airways, and normalization of lungs' tests.

● Chronic bronchitis
- An immediate decrease and, later, elimination of the main symptoms of the disease (cough, dyspnea, heavy breathing, general tiredness, and fatigue).
- Reduction in swelling and hyper-secretion from the mucosal surfaces of bronchi, and elimination of elements of bronchoconstriction.
- Increase in the CP is accompanied by normalization of immunity.
- Prevention of complications (e.g., pneumonia).
- Significant improvements in the quality of life.

● Acute respiratory diseases, including influenza and cold
- Reduction of recovery time from 5-7 days to 1-2 days.
- Prevention of complications (e.g., sinusitis, laryngeal tracheitis, pharingitis, bronchitis, pneumonia, etc.).
- Increase in the CP is accompanied by normalization of immunity.
- Prevention of complications from chronic diseases, such as bronchial asthma, chronic obstructive bronchitis, hypertension, and myocardial ischemia.

● Pneumonia
- An immediate decrease and, later, complete elimination of the main symptoms of the disease (cough and dyspnea) and symptoms of intoxication (general weakness and fatigue).
- Increase in the CP is accompanied by normalization of immunity.
- A decrease in swelling and hyper-secretion of mucus from the bronchi.
- Significant reduction of the time of recovery.

● Rhinitis, sinusitis (frontal sinusitis, metopantritis, maxillary sinusitis)
- Immediate complete or partial restoration of nasal breathing.
- Decrease in doses of vasoconstrictive medications.
- Prevention of appearance of pain and symptoms of intoxication.
- Increase in the CP is accompanied by normalization of immunity and disappearance of inflammatory changes, decrease in swelling and hyper-secretion of mucus from the nasal passages, and decrease in frequency of acute episodes of the disease.
- Surgical interventions become unnecessary.

● Emphysema
- Immediate prevention of progression of the disease, improvement in arterial blood oxygenation tests, and reduction in medication (e.g., cortisol, beta-antagonists, etc.).
- With the increased CP, gradual reduction in production of mucus, if it was present, ability to walk faster with nasal breathing, and improved ability to walk upstairs.
- Use of oxygen 24/7 or lung transplantation becomes unnecessary.
- Years of high CP (about 35 s or more) 24/7 result in gradual regeneration of alveoli and complete restoration of the lungs with normal X-ray results.
- Significant improvements in the quality of life.

Cardiovascular Problems

● Hypertension (primary)
- Immediate elimination of symptoms connected with elevated blood pressure: headache, dizziness, heart palpitations, pain near the heart,

shivering, general fatigue, etc.
- In cases of 1st or 2nd class hypertension, increase in the CP is accompanied by normalization of blood pressure, gradual elimination or significant reduction in doses of medications that reduce blood pressure (or transition from multi-medication to mono-therapy). In cases of 3rd class hypertension, it is possible to significantly reduce medications or make transition to mono-therapy.

- When the CP is 20-30 s or more, the symptoms are absent and no medication is required. This usually takes less than 1-2 months of practice.
- Natural weight normalization.
- Prevention of insulin resistance, diabetes mellitus, hyperlipidemia, and hypertrophy of the left ventricle.
- Prevention of injuries in targeted organs during 1st stage of the disease (myocardial infraction, stroke, angiogenesis of retina, nephropathy, etc.).

• Ischemic heart disease
- Immediate elimination of symptoms of stenocardia attacks (angina pectoris) and prevention of their appearance (or decrease in angina-like pains).
- Increase in the CP is accompanied by transfer from the current functional class of the disease to a less severe one.
- Increase in the CP is accompanied by reduction and elimination of medication (to reduce angina-like pain)
- Significant improvements in the quality of life.

• Heart Failure
- Increase in the CP is accompanied by reduction of the symptoms of chronic cardiac insufficiency (edema of lower extremities, panting, heart palpitations, heartache, general fatigue, tiredness, etc.)
- Increase in the CP is accompanied by decrease in the doses of medications and their number, natural reduction in triglycerides and cholesterol.
- Significant improvements in the quality of life.

• Arrhythmia
- Immediate elimination of heart palpitations and various

accompanying symptoms: unpleasant feelings and pains near the heart, feelings of breathlessness and panting, chill and sweating, general fatigue, etc.

- In cases of chronic forms of tachycardia, increase in the CP is accompanied by steady reduction in the heart rate, recovery of coronary circulation, and perfusion of injured parts of myocardium. That prevents reappearance of paroxysms of pulsating arrhythmia, ventricular tachycardia, etc.

- Significant improvements in the quality of life.

• Varicose veins
- Immediate decrease and, later, elimination of unpleasant symptoms: heaviness and leg cramps, puffiness around the feet, and weakness and fatigue of the lower extremities.
- Increase in the CP is accompanied by decrease in the extent of the capillary bed and enlarged veins.
- Prevention of possible complications due to chronic venous insufficiency: trophic ulcers, thromboembolism, and varicose eczema.
- Significant improvements in the quality of life.

• Dystonia
- Immediate decrease and, later, complete normalization of blood pressure and eliminate various symptoms (sweating, heart palpitations, feelings of inner shivering and obstructed throat, etc.).
- Increase in the CP is accompanied by normalization of emotional life, restoration of sleep, disappearance of pains and aches in various body parts.
- Significant improvements in the quality of life.

Hormonal conditions

• Diabetes mellitus
- Immediate decrease in insulin dosage twofold, use of insulin of short duration.
- Increase in the CP is accompanied by decreased requirements in insulin and, at 35-40 s CP its complete elimination.
- Prevention of complications.

- High CP values (over 35 s) 24/7 lead to complete clinical remission (cure). The time of recovery is usually about 1/10 of the disease time (use of insulin).
- Normalization of the emotional life of the students and significant improvement in the quality of life.

● Hypothyroidism
- Immediate intensification of metabolism, energy level, and reduction in the thyroidal hormone dose
- Increase in the CP is accompanied by increased energy, disappearance of possible feeling cold (e.g., cold extremities) and other negative symptoms.
- High CP values (over 35 s) 24/7 lead to complete clinical remission and no need for medication.
- Prevention of complications.
- Significant improvements in the quality of life.

● Obesity
- Immediate intensification of metabolism and changes in dietary preferences in the direction of "healthier" choices (eating less with better energy).
- Increase in the CP is accompanied by redistribution of fat with its subsequent metabolism and increase in the muscular mass due to the catabolic effect.
- With the increased CP, the ability and desire to exercise is gradually restored. Moreover, use of physical exercise leads to dramatic acceleration of the recovery rate.
- Prevention of complications.
- Significant improvements in the quality of life.

Gastrointestinal problems

● Chronic gastritis
- Immediate decrease and, later, complete elimination of pain and symptoms due to dyspeptic effects (heartburn, regurgitation, nausea, etc.).
- Increase in the CP is accompanied by normalization of colonic tone, phasic contractility of the GI tract, perfusion, metabolic

processes in the mucosal surface of the esophagus and stomach causing accelerated healing of erosions and ulcers, together with regeneration of the mucosal surface of the stomach.
- When the student achieved 35 s morning CP and maintained this level for more than 2 weeks, normalization of the immune profile leads to eradication of Helicobacter Pylori.
- Prevention of complications due to chronic gastritis, and complete clinical remission for many years (cure).
- Significant improvements in the quality of life.

• Chronic non-ulcerative colitis
- Immediate decrease and, later, complete elimination of pain and symptoms due to dyspeptic effects (bloating and rumbling in the belly, regurgitation, nausea, inconsistencies in bowel habits, etc.).
- Increase in the CP is accompanied by normalization of colonic tone, phasic contractility of the GI tract, perfusion, and metabolic processes in the mucosal surface leading to its regeneration.
- When the student achieved 40 s CP or more and maintained this level for more than 2 weeks, normalization of the immune profile leads to normalization of the GI flora with elimination of pathogenic bacteria and inflammation in the lining of the large intestine.
- Prevention of complications.
- Complete clinical remission for many years (cure).
- Significant improvements in the quality of life.

• Chronic pancreatitis
- Immediate decrease and, later, complete elimination of pain and symptoms due to dyspeptic effects (bloating and rumbling in the belly, regurgitation, nausea, vomiting, alternating bowel habits, etc.).
- Increase in the CP is accompanied by normalized colonic tone, phasic contractility of the GI tract and recovered internal secretion.
- Prevention of complications (diabetes mellitus, pancreonecrosis, secondary diseases of the biliary tract, etc.).
- Complete clinical remission for many years (cure).
- Significant improvements in the quality of life.

• Chronic cholecystitis
- Immediate decrease and, later, complete elimination of pain and symptoms due to dyspeptic effects (bloating and rumbling in the

belly, regurgitation, nausea, vomiting, alternating bowel habits, etc.).
- Increase in the CP is accompanied by normalization of colonic tone, phasic
contractility of the GI tract, perfusion, metabolism in the lining of the intestine, tone of the bile-conducting organs and elimination of inflammatory processes in the bile-conducting system.
- When the student achieved 35 s morning CP and maintained this level for more than 2 weeks, normalization of the immune profile leads to normalization of the GI flora, disappearance of pathogenic bacteria and elimination of inflammation in the biliary tract.
- Prevention of complications.
- Inhibition of formation of stones in the gallbladder.
- Complete clinical remission for many years (cure).
- Normalization of the emotional life of the students and significant improvement in the quality of life.

• Gastro-esophageal reflux (GERD)
- Immediate decrease and, later, complete elimination of pain and symptoms due to dyspeptic effects (heartburn and regurgitation).
- Increase in the CP is accompanied by improved perfusion and normalization of the metabolic processes in the mucosal surface of the esophagus and stomach, with accelerated healing of erosions and ulcers.
- When the student achieved 35 s morning CP and maintained this level for more than 2 weeks, normalization of the immune profile leads to normalization of the GI flora, disappearance of pathogenic bacteria and elimination of inflammation in the biliary tract.
- Prevention of recurring appearances of erosions and ulcers.
- Normalization of the emotional life and significant improvement in the quality of life.

Diseases of kidneys and urinary tract

• Chronic pyelonephritis
- Quick elimination of the symptoms (pain and unpleasant sensations during urination, frequent urination, etc.).
- Decrease in the duration of antibacterial therapy and the achievement of positive results using mono-therapy (e.g., use of a

single antibiotic medication).

- In case of chronic states of the disease, the CP growth gradually increases parameters of the immunity.

- Prevention of development of acute complications due to chronic pyelonephritis, and, in future, complete recovery.

- Prevention of more severe forms of pyelonephritis (obstructive urinary pathologies, i.e., urinary stones, polycystic kidney disease, urinary tract reflux, benign prostatic hyperplasia, etc.) and structural changes in the kidneys and urinary tract, as a result of diabetes mellitus, neutropenia, kidney disease, polyarthritis, and other severe conditions.

- Regression of the obstructive effects, pH normalization, prevention of appearance of new stones, and dissolution of old stones and their elimination.

- Significant improvements in the quality of life.

• Kidney and urinary stones

- Quick elimination of the symptoms (pain, unpleasant sensations due to presence of stones in the urinary tract).

- With the increased CP, gradual normalization of the urinary pH, ability to hold more urine without any symptoms, and disappearance of symptoms of the disease

- Prevention of shock wave therapy, surgery, and medication.

- Prevention of complications.

- Significant improvements in the quality of life.

Diseases of the musculoskeletal system

• Osteochondrosis

- Elimination of the symptoms (pain and unpleasant sensations due to bony necrosis).

- With the increased CP, gradual normalization of restorative processes in the affected areas and bone re-growth.

- High CPs (over 35 s) for some weeks result in healing of the bone in a relatively normal shape and absence of any symptoms.

- Prevention of surgery, as in case of Legg-Calvé-Perthes disease, and the need for joint replacement.

- Prevention of complications (e.g., arthritis).

- Significant improvements in the quality of life.

● Polyarthritis
- Immediate reduction or elimination of pain.
- With the increased CP, gradual reduction in joint swelling, and their stiffness and restrictions of movements.
- When the student achieved 35 s morning CP and maintained this level for some weeks, normalization of the regenerative processes in the affected areas leads to elimination of degenerative processes, inflammation, and joint damage and complete disappearance of symptoms.
- Prevention of surgery and the need for joint replacement.
- Prevention of complications.
- Normalization of the emotional life of the students and significant improvements in the quality of life.

● Chronically poor healing of bone fractures
- Immediate reduction or elimination of pain.
- With the increased CP, gradual reduction in possible swelling, stiffness, and restrictions of movements.
- When the student achieved 35 s morning CP and maintained this level for some weeks, normalization of the regenerative processes in the affected areas leads to elimination of degenerative processes, inflammation, and healing of the fracture and complete disappearance of symptoms.
- Prevention of surgery and the need for joint replacement.
- Prevention of complications.
- Significant improvements in the quality of life.

Skin diseases

● Eczema
- Immediate decrease, and with higher CP, total elimination of skin itching.
- Normalization of psychological and emotional states of the student.
- Increase in the CP and its maintenance within 30-40 s range are accompanied by gradual decrease in the area of skin rash with its subsequent complete disappearance.

- Significant improvements in the quality of life.

● Psoriasis
- Immediate decrease, and with higher CP, total elimination of skin itching.
- Normalization of psychological and emotional states of the student.
- Increase in the CP and its maintenance within 30-40 s range are accompanied by gradual decrease in the area of skin rash with its subsequent complete disappearance.
- Prevention of complications (arthropathy, psoriasis erythrodermia, skin infections, amyloidosis, etc.).
- Improvement of the general state of the students (stabilization of the respiratory symptoms of the allergy and the dynamic of the accompanying chronic diseases, i.e. diseases of the GI tract, chronic infections, etc.).
- Significant improvements in the quality of life.

● Neurodermitis
- Immediate decrease, and with higher CP, total elimination of skin itching.
- Normalization of psychological and emotional states of the student.
- Increase in the CP and its maintenance within 30-40 s range are accompanied by gradual decrease in the area of skin rash with its subsequent complete disappearance.
- Restoration of the sleep (in cases of its abnormalities).
- Improvement of the general state of the students (stabilization of the symptoms of the allergy, such as rhinoconjunctivitis, symptoms of bronchial obstruction, etc.).
- Significant improvements in the quality of life.

Allergies and Immunodeficiency

● Allergic rhinitis and nasal polyps
- Immediate restoration of nasal breathing, decrease in nasal discharges, decrease in the dosages and frequency of application of vasoconstrictive medication.
- The growth of the CP is accompanied by stable remission with complete elimination of swelling, medication and full restoration of

nasal breathing.
- Prevention of surgery.
- Normalization of the emotional life of the students and significant improvement in the quality of life.

● Allergic conjunctivitis
- Immediate reduction of symptoms (e.g., itching) and decrease in the amount of medication.
- The growth of the CP is accompanied by complete elimination of skin itching, decrease the area covered with rash, and decrease the duration of use of medication.
- Normalization of the emotional life of the students and significant improvement in the quality of life.

● States of immunodeficiency (secondary)
- Immediate elimination of clinical symptoms of secondary immunodeficiency, such as frequent infective and inflammatory processes in the lungs, bronchi, nasal passages, urinary system, GI tract, eyes, skin, and soft tissues.
- Further CP growth prevents development of similar complications.
- Significant improvements in the quality of life.
- Transition of children and adults from the "frequently sick" category into the "practically healthy" one.

Appendix 4. Typical changes due to the Buteyko breathing exercises and subsequent normalization of breathing

Although the effects of chronic hyperventilation are variable and individual, there are certain changes that are experienced by most people who either normalized their breathing or have made certain progress in this direction. These changes are summarized below.

• Physiological and neurological changes

These changes are based on the more stable autonomic nervous system, with a tendency toward parasympathetic dominance (rather

than the usual stress-induced sympathetic dominance). That usually includes the following changes:
- respiratory efficiency increases (respiratory rate decreases, respiratory amplitude and tidal volume decreases (for the CPs up to 1-2 min), breathing smoothness increases, vital capacity increases, FEV increases)
- cardiovascular efficiency increases (pulse rate and blood pressure decrease)
- electrical skin resistance decreases (less sweating, more relaxation)
- EEG changes: alpha waves increase (theta, delta, and beta waves also increase during various stages of the breathing exercises)
- EMG activity decreases
- gastrointestinal function normalizes (gut flora improves, intestinal tone normalizes, stool consistency improves, bowel movements become easier and more regular, constipation disappears)
- skin gets stronger, shining, more resilient and elastic (sebaceous glands produce more oil); skin rashes, skin sagging, easy skin bruising, skin dryness and noxious sweat odor disappear; wound healing time is decreased
- skin flora, skin respiration, skin sensations, and skin excretory functions improve
- wound-healing time and accompanied inflammation around wounds decrease
- water balance and kidney function improve (less water is required for proper hydration, urinary frequency decreases and urinary volume increases, puffiness and excessive water retention disappears)
- various endocrine functions normalize (energy level increases, weight normalizes, appetite improves)
- sleeping quality improves (less time is required for falling asleep; sleeping time is decreased; more time is spent in deep, dreamless sleep; the number of awakenings is smaller (down to 0 when the CP is above 60 s); less or no discomfort or pain is experienced; the number of body's movements and changing positions during the sleep is decreased [down to 0])
- musculoskeletal and joint flexibility increases
- posture improves
- strength and resiliency increase
- endurance increases

- immunity increases
- pain threshold increases.

• General psychological and social changes

Psychological changes are manifested in more efficient work of the nervous system and permanent changes in personal attitudes towards surrounding environment, self, and other people. These changes are possible due to increased blood supply to the brain (section 1.4) and increased threshold of neuronal excitability (also section 1.4). The person has an increased ability to remain calm under stressful conditions. Among these are the following changes:
- anxiety and depression decrease, mood swings disappear
- well-being increases
- self-acceptance and self-actualization increase
- cognitive function and perception improve
- attention, concentration, memory (both, short and long-term), learning efficiency, and various logical abilities improve
- more objective perceptions of the outside world, other people, own place in this world, and own abilities and limitations are possible
- hostility decreases
- tolerance and social adjustment increases
- addictions, cravings, and unhealthy attachments disappear
- the desire to find the truth and essence of objects, processes and activities increases.

• Biochemical effects

Normalization of various biochemical processes is revealed in the following changes (these are confirmed by blood analysis):
- blood glucose and insulin levels decrease, insulin sensitivity increases
- plasma sodium decreases
- total cholesterol decreases (triglycerides decrease, HDL cholesterol increases, LDL cholesterol decreases, VLDL cholesterol decreases, cholinesterase increases)
- thyroxin level and ATPase increase
- hematocrit and hemoglobin level increase

- lymphocyte count increases, total white blood cell count decreases
- total serum protein increases.

• Technical skills

Changes in technical skills are possible due to better communication between the nervous system and muscles. Various technical and psychomotor functions improve, including:
- dexterity and fine motor skills
- grip strength
- eye-hand coordination
- reaction time and choice reaction time
- steadiness and balance
- execution of complicated movements.

• Changes in physical and general sport skills

Psychology-related and physiology-related changes are also manifested in improvements in various physical and sport skills. They are based on domination of subcortical regions of the brain and domination of the parasympathetic part of the autonomic nervous system. These changes are in comparison with previous states (corresponding to chronic hyperventilation) during similar physical exercise. It can be noticed and often measured that now the person has:
- more accurate and goal-oriented movements (in the past, the movements during the periods of depression were too slow, while during excitements and bursts of activities were too fast and imprecise)
- normalization of muscle tone
- lower risk of injuring muscles and ligaments
- lower energy spending (efforts are minimum, irrelevant muscles and the rest of the body are more relaxed, activity of opposing muscle groups is more balanced)
- increased maximum oxygen uptake
- increased maximum tolerated lactate level
- non-competitive, goal-oriented, more detached and objective attitude.

Recommended reading

To learn and/or refine your Buteyko breathing exercises, consider this 2013 Amazon book (Kindle and paperback): "Advanced Buteyko Breathing Exercises" - http://www.amazon.com/Advanced-Buteyko-Breathing-Exercises-ebook/dp/B00CAXAKAA/. It considers, in detail, many unique topics and effects that are not present in any other book.

Do you know that, in relation to foods and diets, it is more important what eats you rather than a modern obsession with "you are what you eat"? There are clear and specific numerous signs of ideal or normal digestion, which include a clean tongue (no white or yellow coating to scrape) and no need to use toilet paper (no soiling). If soiling is present, that means that one has poor GI flora, and this reduces body oxygenation and reduces your CP during sleep. The PDF book "Perfect Digestion" deals with these symptoms and explains how to achieve no soiling and other signs of great GI health. You can get this book from NormalBreathing site: How to Improve Digestion with Lifestyle and Higher Body O2 - http://www.normalbreathing.com/how-to/how-to-improve-digestion.php or go on Smashwords where you can find many other formats (such as EPUB, Kindle, LRF, PDB, etc.) "Perfect Digestion" - https://www.smashwords.com/books/view/327725

Please, feel free to leave you honest review on the Amazon page of this book.

Printed in Great Britain
by Amazon